CLASSROOM YOGA BREAKS

Norton Books in Education

CLASSROOM YOGA BREAKS

Brief Exercises to Create Calm

Louise Goldberg

W.W. Norton & Company
Independent Publishers Since 1923
New York • London

For information about permission to reproduce selections from this book, write to Permissions, W. W. Norton & Company, Inc., 500 Fifth Avenue, New York, NY 10110

For information about special discounts for bulk purchases, please contact W. W. Norton Special Sales at specialsales@wwnorton.com or 800-233-4830

Manufacturing by RR Donnelley Willard
Production manager: Chris Critelli

Library of Congress Cataloging-in-Publication Data

Names: Goldberg, Louise, 1950– author.
Title: Classroom yoga breaks : brief exercises to create calm / Louise
  Goldberg.
Description: First edition. | New York : W.W Norton & Company, [2017] |
  Includes bibliographical references and index.
Identifiers: LCCN 2016015309 | ISBN 9780393710953 (hardcover)
Subjects: LCSH: Classroom management. | Hatha yoga for children.
Classification: LCC LB3013 .G628 2017 | DDC 371.102/4—dc23 LC record
available at https://lccn.loc.gov/2016015309

ISBN: 978-0-393-71095-3

W. W. Norton & Company, Inc., 500 Fifth Avenue, New York, N.Y. 10110
                www.wwnorton.com
W. W. Norton & Company Ltd., 15 Carlisle Street, London W1D 3BS

1 2 3 4 5 6 7 8 9 0

To my teacher JoAnn Evans, for your friendship and example

To my son Mark Goldberg-Foss, for making me laugh and think

And to my husband Rich Foss, for being there for me, always

Contents

Acknowledgments

M Y THANKS TO all the students and teachers whose photos grace this book, and especially to the families who granted me permission to share their children's talents.

I am indebted to my photographer and friend Ed Zeiss for his extraordinary eye, his patience and gentleness with the children, and his willingness to always go the extra mile. And to my friend and fellow yoga teacher Bryna Cain, for her stellar photography, including the cover and author photos. She made each photo shoot into a joyful occasion for the children and me. As you'll see, Ed and Bryna's work brings this text to life.

I was flabbergasted when Deborah Malmud, my editor at W. W. Norton, contacted me about writing my first book, *Yoga Therapy for Children with Autism and Special Needs*. In fact, I wondered if she had reached the right person. I still cherish my copy of *The Norton Anthology of English Literature* from my college years, and my husband and I have a shelf full of Norton texts. Once I got over the shock, I couldn't wait to begin.

When she proposed this project, however, I didn't feel ready to write another book. Having done it once and discovered the magnitude of the task, I was reluctant to begin again. The importance of this subject, however, rendered my concerns inconsequential. It is because of Deborah's encouragement, vision, and ability to make an enormous project seem doable that this book has come to be.

My thanks to Alison Lewis whose editorial commentary and organizational suggestions were extremely helpful. Elizabeth Baird oversaw the production of the book, crafting the beautiful product that you now hold. Thanks to Kevin Olsen and the marketing group at Norton for their diligence. Becoming a Norton author has been like winning the lottery. I am grateful to this extraordinary team of professionals who truly care about books and their authors. Thanks to Karen Fisher for her copyediting skills and Sheryl Rowe for taking exquisite care with composition and coaching me through the final stages of the book.

I'd like to thank my teachers, students, family, and friends for their gracious support and encouragement throughout the writing process. I am grateful to my yoga community, especially my longtime friend and teacher JoAnn Evans, whose knowledge and love for yoga infuse my teaching and to Eunice Wellington for her inspiration. Thank you to my first teachers: Carole Goya, Swami Vishnudevananda, and Pearl Van Aalst.

My gratitude to the students and faculty of the Yoga Center of Deerfield Beach, Florida, my spiritual home, and especially to our director, Dotty Zevin, for her unflagging support and encouragement to "fly."

Two friends reviewed the entire text: My yoga student Susan Vladeck whose editing skills have been honed assisting her talented children, and my longtime friend Barbara Harris, retired English teacher and librarian, who has a knack for cutting excess. Thanks to them and massage therapist Jody Kenyon for her thoughtful input on my stress chapter.

Thanks to my friends and family who propped me up when I needed it: my sister Roberta Callaghan, who knew when to listen and when to "let me go"; acupuncture physician Steve Templin and psychotherapist Eileen Templin, who shared ideas about the brain, stress, and learning; Wilma Schiller for discussing respiration; Karen Deerwester, author and teacher, for inspiring me with her own work; Debby Reynolds, Joni and Pat Clare, Brenda Martin, Marty O'Neill, Kathy Hurley, Howard and Anita Goldberg, and Siri Goldberg. Thanks to you all for knowing when to talk and when to leave me alone.

Thanks to my partners in *S.T.O.P. and Relax© Your Special Needs Yoga Toolbox*—Debra Collins, Daniela Morales, and Sally Miller—for pooling their talents to bring a visual yoga-based curriculum to children in schools around the world.

My gratitude to John Smith, retired principal, who introduced the yoga program to the Broward Schools in 1981, and to Sally Creswell, retired curriculum coordinator, who continued the project with autism education in 2000.

I was fortunate to have the opportunity to visit a number of schools while doing research for this project. A very special thank you goes to the Broward County Public Schools, especially to GiGi McIntire, the administration, and faculty at Mirror Lakes Elementary School for their extraordinary contributions to this book. Thanks to Machiko Morishita-Horner and the administration of Dania Elementary School. Thank you to Sondra Sellitti of Monarch High for testing out some of the BREATHE FIRST lessons with her classes and to Renae Lapin for brainstorming with me.

My thanks to middle school principal Patrice Rogers and to yoga teacher Pam Leal for letting me observe school yoga classes at North Broward Prep. I am indebted to Stefanie Gross who gave me a whole day to observe Move Through Yoga classes at Atlantic West High and Boca Raton High of the Palm Beach School District and to Principal Geoff McKee and teacher Catherine Freihofer for speaking with me about the program. I am grateful to Nancy Lieberman, Stacy Layer, and the remarkable faculty of Baudhuin Preschool of Nova Southeastern University for implementing S.T.O.P. and Relax yoga into their curriculum. Special thanks to Donna Davis for welcoming me into her dance kinetics classes at Edgewater High School in Orlando, Florida, for sharing her passion, and for becoming a friend.

I am grateful to my colleague and friend Sharon Trull for transporting me and permitting me to follow her through a day of teaching Yoga 4 Classrooms at a New Hampshire elementary school, and to Cathy Calandriello for speaking with me and inviting me to observe her and Stacey McDonough teaching yoga at Dover Middle School.

Thanks to Sat Bir Khalsa and Bethany Butzer for their tireless research on school yoga and for making that material available to me. I am indebted to my friend Lisa Flynn of ChildLight Yoga for welcoming me into the national school yoga community and to Karma Lynn Carpenter for selflessly championing this movement. I am grateful to them and to the extraordinary group of visionaries and leaders in the field of school yoga and mindfulness, who so generously gave their time to be interviewed for this book: Ali Smith, Allison Morgan, Allyson Copacino, Anne Desmond, Beth Johnson, Brynne Caleda, Carla Tantillo-Philibert, Catherine Cook-Cottone, Caverly Morgan, Cheryl Crawford, Chris Theodore, Debby Kaminsky, Hannah Gould, Haris Lender, Iona Smith, Joanne Spence, Jodi Komitor, Katherine Ghannam, Kathy Flaminio, Kelli Love, Laura Rubenstein,

Lynea Gillam, Marissa Lipovsky, and Terri Cooper. Thanks for input from Andrea Hyde, Anne Buckley-Reem, Craig Hanauer, Don and Marsha Wenig, Jennifer Cohen Harper, and Laura Douglass.

Thank you to the educators and researchers who graciously responded to my questions: Steven Porges, Jaak Panksepp, Beth Navon, Carla Barrett, Cynthia Zurchin, Mark Greenberg, Patricia Jennings, Patricia Broderick, Audrey R. Tyrka, Clinton Lewis, Brian Chatard, Jennifer Frank, Katherine Weare, Deb Stone, and Dolly Lambdin.

I am grateful for permission to share material from Amy Weintraub, the Himalayan Institute of Yoga Science and Philosophy, Kripalu Yoga in the Schools Teacher Training, and Dr. Steven Templin. Special thanks for the contributions from Angela Van Hemert, Michael Comfort, Jeremy Cain, Rosana Giani, Julia Barber, Meg Webb, and Roja Pendakur.

I am grateful to the many students, clients, and friends who graciously supported my preoccupation with this book, including Beth and Dick Heath, Bonny Palmer, Chrissy Hansen, Brigitte Galinkin, Dan Ewing, Fran Mulcahy, Joyce Marando, Kimberly Ferrara, Linda Becker, Marie Zappala-Stewart, Tina Kaplan, and Norma Abrahams, and to my Aunt Janet Skolnik for cheering me on.

Thanks to Bill Longstreth, Roy Feifer, and my dear friend Elizabeth McKay, for keeping me healthy during this demanding stretch.

I am grateful to my son, Mark Goldberg-Foss, musician, historian, activist, for his good humor, kindness, and the inspiration of his inquiring mind.

To my husband and partner Rich Foss, for reading, rereading, editing, cooking, cleaning, encouraging, commiserating, clarifying, listening, and supporting me through every phase of this process. How fortunate I am to have you in my life.

And to our dog Ralph, for teaching us about the process of aging with grace.

Finally, I want to thank my parents Abe and Annette Goldberg for creating and nurturing our wonderful tribe: my siblings Howard, Steve, and Roberta; grandchildren Michael, Eric, Siri, Sarah, Rachel, Rebecca, Mark; 13 great-grandchildren and their families. How proud they would be of all of you! We were blessed to have had parents who instilled in each of their children and grandchildren a belief in ourselves, in one another, and in the natural goodness of others. I wish they were here to share this moment.

Introduction

AFTER TEACHING HIGH school English and remedial reading at the middle school level in New England, I moved to Florida in the late 1970s. Shortly thereafter I began teaching English as an adjunct faculty member at a small local college. The college provisionally accepted any high school graduate and offered remedial courses as needed for students to qualify for matriculation. I taught remedial composition to students, many of whom worked full or part time to support families while tackling college. It always struck me as particularly onerous that these students had to master a skill that they had already struggled with in high school—while paying for the privilege.

About one-third of my students never completed the course. One young man in particular caught my attention. Jeremy was bright and articulate. He could explain himself clearly verbally, but as soon as I handed him a piece of paper to convey the same thoughts, his eyes widened in terror, his breathing became erratic, and his palms so sweaty that he had difficulty holding a pen. A strong young man who could have outrun and out-lifted anyone in the class, Jeremy was immobilized by this task. It was a huge disappointment to me when he dropped the course, because I knew he couldn't continue his college education without it. My inability to support him troubled me, and I was determined to find more resources for students like him in the future.

During this period, personal transitions and family losses had led me to my first yoga class. It was love from the start. My practice had become increasingly important in managing stress and improving my overall fitness.

In the summer of 1981, I completed my yoga teacher training at the Sivananda Yoga Camp in Val Morin, just north of Montreal. Living in a pup tent on the side of a mountain in the Laurentians, arising each morning at 5:00 for meditation, I spent full days studying philosophy and Sanskrit and practicing postures and breathing exercises. For a month, I trekked up the mountain by flashlight each night after evening meditation. All this was fueled by two vegan meals each day.

Upon completion of my training, I had the opportunity to teach yoga as an adjunct in the Physical Education (PE) Department, at the same college where I was teaching English. My colleague Carole Goya and I developed and taught introductory yoga classes. By student request, the college added advanced courses.

Most of my PE students were freshmen, and almost none of them had experienced yoga before. I started with the gentlest of postures and breathing techniques, and moved gradually into more advanced variations of each. The class met for 2.5 hours twice a week; it was a delight to watch the students gain flexibility, balance, and strength throughout the semester. While my English students sweated and struggled over their writing assignments, my PE students grew gradually more relaxed and self-confident, willing to face new challenges each week.

While my experiences on the two sides of the campus—English and PE departments—were vastly different, I began to wonder if and how they might overlap.

In my yoga classes, I began to coach students to incorporate yoga techniques into daily activities in school or at home. We worked with breathing techniques that could be useful in challenging social situations. I reinforced methods for improving mental focus in academic classes. We discussed positive attitude and practiced quiet sitting in meditation and progressively relaxing body and mind. One of my students, a slender young redhead, came to me after class one day, close to tears. She told me that she had suffered with severe asthma her entire life, and described some of the ways it had inhibited her as an athlete and an otherwise free-spirited child. For as long as she could remember, whenever she struggled to breathe, someone would tell her to relax and take a deep breath. "Try to relax when you can't breathe," she laughed. "And the more I panicked because I couldn't calm down, the more breathless I became. In 19 years of struggling with this condition, it wasn't until now, through yoga, that anyone ever taught me *how* to relax" (Goldberg, 2004b, p. 71).

A bright young man named Alex proudly informed me that he had finally passed his public speaking class—the last requirement for his associate's degree. Now he could continue his studies at the university where he had been accepted. In the past, he explained, "Whenever I would stand up to speak, even though I knew the speech cold, I would freeze and nothing would come out. Not a sound." This had happened three times. But toward the end of his second semester practicing yoga, he approached his speech teacher for one last opportunity. "I still felt the panic and restriction in my chest," he confessed, "but I breathed and told myself that I was calm, focused. I slowed down my mind, and the words tumbled out. I'm not saying it was a great speech, but I did it!"

In fact, the most consistent improvement shared by my yoga PE students at the end of each semester was in the area of public speaking. The ability to breathe, to self-calm, and to retain their focus was positively affecting their ability to express themselves in their academic classes. They talked about greater patience with others in classes, at home, and on the highway, better eating habits, sounder sleep, and an overall improved sense of well-being.

Having seen the varied areas of change that my students credited to their yoga practice, I began to wonder if the flip side of this equation might work. Would bringing a bit of yoga into my academic classes, in the form of a warm-up at the beginning of class or a break between activities, have a positive effect on the students in my composition classes? I experimented with shoulder shrugs and neck rolls before writing assignments. Then I added some simple breathing practices at the beginning of class. Although my students thought I was weird, they were willing to give it a try. Instead of the deer-in-the-headlights look that I had been getting when giving a classroom writing assignment, students shrugged their shoulders a few times, took several deep breaths, and got to it. When they came to my office with frustrations and questions, we'd take a deep breath together before and during the explanation process. As their emotional short fuses lengthened, their attention spans appeared to lengthen. At the very least, they were completing assignments and staying on task.

I wish I could tell you that they all became proficient writers. Some of them struggled with this basic skill throughout the course, and perhaps throughout their college careers. Nonetheless, learning to regulate their anxiety through simple yoga techniques was enough to give some of these students a chance, maybe their first chance, to succeed.

This early 1980s experiment became the origin of Creative Relaxation, my approach to implementing yoga-based techniques in classrooms for students of varied needs.

What You Will Find in the Pages Ahead

This book is divided into five sections, beginning with an explanation of what yoga is. Chapter 1 explores yoga from its origins thousands of years ago to its current inclusion by the National Institutes of Health as a leading complementary therapy. Chapter 2 provides an overview of yoga for schools—how and why it belongs in schools, the research summarizing its efficacy, and an introduction to the school yoga movement.

Part II examines the many school needs that yoga addresses. In Chapter 3, we consider how it complements mindfulness training, which often includes yoga postures, breathing exercises, and meditation. Chapter 4 enumerates ways that yoga complements social and emotional learning (SEL), as described by Collaborative for Academic, Social, and Emotional Learning. Self-awareness and self-management, for example, are SEL competencies that are enhanced by yoga practices such as focused breathing and tension release techniques. Chapter 5 discusses yoga as a noncompetitive fitness regimen that is complementary to the objectives of school PE programs. The growing role of yoga among professional and amateur athletes is also considered here. The use of yoga exercises school-wide and in small groups for Response to Intervention and Positive Behavioral Interventions and Supports is discussed in Chapter 6. Bullying is a topic of great concern to many educators. Yoga's role as an intervention for bullying behaviors is investigated in Chapter 7. The subject of Chapter 8 is yoga's efficacy for students with autism spectrum disorder and other special needs. This touches upon some of the topics covered in my book *Yoga Therapy for Children with Autism and Special Needs* (Goldberg, 2013), such as the importance of visual cues, the challenge of touch sensitivity, and how to set a mood for relaxation. Tools for improving focus and self-calming are introduced here. The final consideration in Part II is the importance of developing a partnership with the school community when bringing yoga into its curriculum. Suggestions for working with administrators, teachers, and parents are included in Chapter 9.

Part III explores the relationship between yoga and neuroscience. If you are interested in research, this section will intrigue you. Otherwise, you might skim the chapters for those topics that are pertinent to your students and your program. Chapter 10 examines the body's response to stress and how it affects students' behavior and capacity to absorb information. Fascinating research on the development of the adolescent brain is useful in understanding why breathing practices and movement, for example, are often useful strategies for relieving teen anxiety. The benefits of exercise relative to learning and the perils of its absence are discussed in Chapter 11. Using research and anecdotal reports from varied school yoga programs, Chapter 12 explores yoga's role in improving students' capacity for self-control. Its function in increasing resilience and redirecting troubled youth supports the case for yoga's inclusion in varied educational settings. Chapter 13 delves into the research that correlates yoga with improved executive function. Self-control, working memory, mental flexibility, and sustained attention have been shown to contribute to academic and social success—all supported through the practice of yoga.

The fourth part presents the application of yoga for school settings through the principles of Creative Relaxation. I began developing my program for school yoga in the early 1980s, and it has led me to write this book. Chapter 14 introduces the first principle: creating an environment where your students feel safe. You will learn techniques for promoting quiet in your classroom and setting a peaceful mood through breathing and movement. The second principle of Creative Relaxation, engaging the student, is considered in Chapter 15. Having fun and moving together builds connections. Through yoga breaks, you can model kindness and promote a more compassionate experience among your students. In Chapter 16, we examine ways to promote success within your classroom. Suggestions are offered here for implementing yoga breaks to help students better use their time and to improve their ability to attend. The final chapter in Part IV focuses on autonomy. Yoga breaks in the school day foster independence by providing outlets for frustration. Postures are effective for improving body awareness and teaching students how to set personal boundaries.

Part V provides a complete curriculum for implementing brief yoga breaks in your school or classroom. The BREATHE FIRST Yoga and Mindfulness Curriculum includes each of these elements: movement, breathing exercises, relaxation, and mindful awareness practices. The 12 units within the curriculum are arranged by theme, with lessons consisting of 1- to 5-minute exercises for use in academic classrooms.

Each unit includes classroom activities related to the theme, including topics for writing or discussion, breathing exercises, yoga movements that can be done from the seat or standing, focusing exercises to improve attention skills, and relaxation practices. The lessons are illustrated with multiple photographs. Descriptions are provided for each posture in language that is suitable for you to use when instructing your students.

Each unit is designed to expand on a theme, derived from the acronym BREATHE FIRST: B, breathing; R, relaxation; E, exercise; A, attention; T, tuning in and tuning out; H, heart opening; E, expressing; F, fun; I, intention; R, reset; S, sense of self; T, in touch.

You may select complete lessons or single breathing exercises or yoga poses from each lesson. The curriculum contains more than enough material for daily or weekly yoga breaks throughout the semester or school year.

The appendixes deal with self-care. They offer independent practices for teachers in school or at home. During your prep time or lunch break, you can sit at your desk or kick off your shoes to work out some tension. Students will find at-home routines as well as a questionnaire designed to help them select their own yoga breaks. Finally, there are warm-up and cool-down routines to augment PE classes and a core strength routine recommended by a professional football player.

My great hope in writing this book is to inspire you to incorporate yoga breaks in your classroom, so that school becomes a place of healing as well as learning—for you and your students.

PART I

WHAT IS YOGA?

Yoga is a movement therapy that teaches children how to quiet and focus their minds. It builds strength, flexibility, and balance and improves a child's capacity to perceive and interact within the world; breathing techniques calm the mind and still the body. Through mindfulness and one-pointedness, the child develops self-awareness. Creative play . . . and partner interaction make yoga . . . fun. Children stretch their imaginations as they stretch their bodies. Yoga is noncompetitive; partnering in poses and sharing thoughts create a sense of community and elevate self-esteem. (Goldberg, 2013, p. 18)

CHAPTER 1

Building Your Yoga House

Origins of Yoga

Have you heard the tale of the five blind men who are asked to describe an elephant? One man, touching its ear, says the elephant is silky smooth. Another, standing near its foot, describes it as solid as stone. The one at the tusk says it's sharp. The man at the trunk likens the elephant to a tree branch. Feeling its belly, the last man declares the elephant wrinkled and soft. Each one mistakenly generalizes one aspect of the great beast as its complete identity.

Yoga has also been described in many ways. To some it's a form of exercise—rigorous, moderate, or gentle. Others consider it a system of breathing. There are students whose focus is primarily meditation. Some are interested in the healing properties of diet and lifestyle. Study of ancient texts or chant may call others to yoga. Children's yoga is playful and interactive, often including songs and games as well as instruction in acceptance and compassion for others.

There are practitioners who dazzle fans at yoga exhibitions, much like Cirque du Soleil. Many people do yoga while seated in chairs, and some from hospital

3

beds. Others combine laughter with yoga breathing and movement. Yoga therapy is a healing modality, addressing specific symptoms in an effort to improve overall well-being (International Association of Yoga Therapists, 2012).

For many, yoga class is comparable to going to the gym—a place to sweat and move to music. Others consider it a personal, even spiritual practice. Public school yoga is a secular system, void of religious practices. Like the blind men and the elephant, we would be remiss to describe yoga as just one of these things. In fact, the word "yoga," which comes from the Sanskrit root "yuj, to yoke," is often translated as "union" (Feuerstein, 1997, p. 342). At the Sivananda Yoga ashrams and centers where I took much of my training, instruction includes "proper exercise, proper breathing, proper relaxation, proper diet, positive thinking (deep philosophy) and meditation" (Vishnudevananda, 1960, p. xi). My teacher, Swami Vishnudevananda, believed that students enter yoga through many doorways; he welcomed them all, exactly as they were.

Yoga is a systematic approach to well-being, self-regulation, and responsible social interactions. Through exercise, breathing practices, relaxation, mindful practices, and meditation, yoga enhances physical, mental, and emotional health and fitness. It offers tools for developing "happiness, a calm mind, abundant vitality, concentration of genius" (Easwaran, 2007, p. 47). Described as "skill in action" (Gandhi, 2000, p. 49), yoga teaches the most economical ways to use muscular and mental energy, and techniques for discharging that effort when it is no longer needed.

People have been practicing aspects of yoga for over 5,000 years (Easwaran, 2007). Some scholars say yoga may be 8,000 years old. The teachings were passed on by spoken word for millennia. Finally, about 2,000 years ago, yoga instruction was organized into a guidebook called the *Yoga Sutra* (Feuerstein, 1998) by an Indian teacher named Patanjali. In this very short text, Patanjali synthesized all those years of instruction into eight rungs or steps to follow for attaining a calm, quiet mind.

There have been countless translations of the *Yoga Sutra* in dozens of languages (White, 2014). Patanjali's second verse (1.2) is routinely recited by yoga teachers in classes around the world today: "Yoga chitta vrtti nirodah," translated as, "Yoga is the control of thought-waves in the mind" (Prabhavananda & Isherwood, 1981, p. 15).

A yoga posture or asana is defined by Patanjali as a steady, comfortable seated position, practiced in a relaxed state (Feuerstein, 1997). The text instructs practitioners to sit upright with the spine aligned, to facilitate respiration, focus, and concentration.

While most people think of yoga as a series of exercises to twist, stretch, and turn the body upside down, the varied postures that are familiar today are a relatively new aspect of this ancient system. From the *Hatha Yoga Pradipika*, written in the mid-14th century (Feuerstein, 1997), these poses provide additional tools for building strength, increasing flexibility, improving balance, and fostering tranquility. Eunice Wellington, one of my longtime teachers, was a stickler for precision in posture. Yet she described the most advanced asana as "one in which all effort has ceased"—finding effortlessness in the pose. The primary purpose of all these postures is to prepare the body to sit in stillness, move with ease, and experience inner calm.

Although the rungs or steps of yoga, as described by Patanjali, are often practiced separately, each is important. The first rung includes guidelines for getting along with others, such as kindness and truthfulness. This is followed by personal practices like cleanliness and moderation. The third step includes yoga postures to make the body strong and supple. Next is breathing, which can be calming or energizing, and helps the student observe the activity of the mind. Fifth is focus, learning to perceive sources of distraction and finding tools to redirect the mind. The next practice is concentration—on the breath or an object such as a candle flame or flower. This prepares the student for the seventh rung, to sit quietly in meditation, defined as extended concentration. The final rung of Patanjali's teachings, similar to the fifth pillar in Abraham Maslow's (1999) hierarchy of needs, is an experience of unity or wholeness.

Many systems of yoga focus primarily on asanas, yoga postures. Others make ethical living their priority. Stress reduction and relaxation are emphasized in many programs; others work more with breathing or focusing exercises as preparation for meditation. School yoga, as we will explore in Chapter 2, is a secular system of movement, breathing, relaxation, and focusing exercises to improve learning readiness. Any or all of these practices constitute yoga.

> **Qualities of a Yoga Student**
>
> Not agitating the world or by it agitated, he stands above the sway of elation, competition, and fear . . . is friendly and compassionate . . . looks upon friend and foe with equal regard . . . is not buoyed up by praise nor cast down by blame . . . but lets things come and go as they happen. (Easwaran, 2007, p. 208–209)

Yoga Today

Since 2002, yoga has consistently ranked one of the top 10 complementary health approaches used in the United States, according to the National Institutes of Health (NIH). Yoga, a "meditative movement practice used for health purposes, . . . combines physical postures, breathing techniques, and meditation or relaxation" (NCCIH, June, 2013).

> The 2015 National Health Statistics Report on the use of complementary and alternative therapies is based on surveys of nearly 90,000 individuals in 2012. They reported an increase in the practice of yoga across all ages, races, and ethnicities in the United States.
>
> Yoga among adults:
>
> - 21 million adults practice yoga
> - Ages 18–44 increased practice by nearly 50% since 2002
> - Ages 45–64 increased practice from 5.2% to 7.2% since 2002 (Clark et al., 2015)
>
> Yoga among children ages 4–17:
>
> - 1.7 million children practice yoga
> - 400,000 more children practicing in 2012 than 2007
> - Overall increase from 2.3% in 2007 to 3.1% in 2012 (Black et al., 2015)

Numerous benefits for adult practitioners have now been documented. Yoga has been shown to reduce anxiety (Kirkwood et al., 2005), increase pain tolerance (Villemure et al., 2013), and improve sleep (Khalsa, 2004). Studies show that yoga can elevate mood and ease symptoms of post-traumatic stress disorder (PTSD) (Streeter et al., 2010), as well as improve overall quality of life (Woodyard, 2011). A clinical research review cites evidence that yoga improves musculoskeletal and neurological disorders in addition to immune problems (Field, 2011). Research has revealed lower performance anxiety among young adult musicians who practice yoga and meditation (Khalsa et al., 2009) and decreased depressive symptoms among young adults (Woolery et al., 2004).

Scientists have fMRI documentation that meditation alters the structure of the brain, thickening areas that generally thin with age (Lazar et al., 2005), increasing the number of cells in the area of the brain that improves memory (Hölzel et al., 2011), and decreasing the number of cells in the area where anger registers (Hölzel et al., 2011). Yoga has been shown to increase problem-solving abilities and brain functional organization (Gard, Taquet, et al., 2014).

Building Your Yoga House

In some ways, practicing yoga is like building your very own house. You start at the bottom to lay the foundation. Methodically, you work your way up to the upper floors and roof. The materials for the foundation are solid and strong. They need to be so that your structure is sound. As you move up to the top, the materials are more variable and less constant. In yoga, this is called moving from dense to subtle.

Yoga's foundation consists of ethical social practices that affect how you interact with others. When you're building a house, you're going to need assistance; it's too big a job to do alone. And if you're going to live amicably with the people in your neighborhood, you'll need to adhere to certain precepts for how to get along without harming others (or yourself). The first layer in the foundation of your yoga house will be treating others with kindness, being truthful, respecting others' property, using energy wisely, and not being greedy.

The second phase of building your yoga house includes self-awareness practices. If you're going to all the trouble of building a house, it makes sense to commit to taking care of it. These practices are cleanliness, gratitude, self-discipline, self-awareness, and the capacity for acceptance. No matter how extravagant or how modest your house, these principles will determine the quality of your personal life within your home.

The third step requires plying the building materials, in this case the body, to make it sturdy, flexible, and stable. This is the rung of yoga that most are familiar with—exercises and postures. Your house needs to be strong enough to withstand gusty winds and pelting rain, yet pliable enough to adapt to extreme heat and cold. All of the building materials must be aligned and stacked in just the right way to keep your house upright, much like your spinal column keeps you standing up straight.

Now you are ready for the fourth rung in the building of your yoga house. This involves laying the pipes and wiring. You want to choose the best-quality materials available so they will last for the long haul. Here you make choices about the kinds of fuel you will use to keep your home cool in summer and warm in winter. This will affect your comfort throughout all the seasons. Your body is fueled and purified through the process of respiration. Inhalation is the intake of oxygen and other essential gases and exhalation the release of carbon dioxide and other waste. Yoga breathing can be cooling or warming, calming or energizing, as long as it is practiced with awareness.

In the fifth phase of construction, you define the structure of the house, distinguishing outside from inside. You insert doors and windows to make your empty space useful. Still aware of everything that's outside, you begin turning your focus inward to construct the inner dwelling.

Now that you have windows in your house, it's awfully tempting to keep looking outside at the sky and trees. But you still have lots to do before your house is complete. The walls and ceilings need painting; the flooring must be finished. Redirection of the mind is not always easy. Returning your attention to this inner space is called concentration. This sixth rung requires increased focus and self-awareness, so you can see why those qualities of self-discipline introduced in the second rung are essential from the start.

Next you can begin bringing in furniture, hanging pictures, and decorating the rooms the way you want them to be. All of this work leads to the seventh rung of construction. This is the phase that most homeowners long for—creating a haven where you can sit, relax, and simply be. Free from judgment and distraction, content and comfortable, you find the stillness within your own home. This is the practice of meditation.

Having taken all these building materials and made this space truly your own—a place to be yourself and still feel connected to others—at last you can sit on your own back porch. Resting in your favorite lounge chair, overlooking the neighborhood, you feel a sense of community. Your neighbors walk past. Some wave and smile; others don't look your way. Although each is different from you in some ways, there is harmony and mutual acceptance. This is union, the connection among all beings, the final rung of yoga.

The yoga house is one that you build using your own body and mind, so it's more portable than the structure that you may inhabit today. This is the inner home that you carry with you— and carries you— throughout your entire life.

Let's begin!

CHAPTER 2

Yoga for Schools Overview

BEING A STUDENT is stressful. Pressure to succeed starts in the early grades and escalates through high school. With budgetary constraints and increased emphasis on core competencies and test preparation, elective classes are often cut or underfunded. Physical education (PE) classes have been eliminated from many elementary schools. Middle and high school PE classes are often extremely large, with fewer staff and resources to equip their programs. Funding and insurance constraints have led many schools to eliminate field trips, pep rallies, parties, and dances. As a result, going to school is a lot less fun for many children.

Competition for class rank and college admission, continual distractions by technology, increased emphasis on high-stakes testing, and the pressure to act and look more like adults than they are prepared to be often lead to confusion for students. Bullying, anger and depression, obesity and body image issues, gang affiliations, and violence can overshadow a school's mission to educate youth. These factors contribute to an environment where fear and anxiety are often the impetus for a young person's choices and behaviors.

Teachers, too, reflect the pressures of addressing larger classes, more diverse learning styles within their classrooms, increased demands for accountability, and feeling less safe within their schools.

There is no single or simple solution to these varied challenges. Many schools are implementing photo IDs and security cameras to keep students under continual surveillance. Others use metal detectors and armed guards to prevent intruders and students from bringing weapons onto campus. Hopefully, these efforts will succeed in making schools safer. But even a secure building does not guarantee that students feel safe. Without the skills to reduce anxiety and focus the mind, school becomes another source of untenable stress.

Yoga helps create a safe space for students and teachers. By empowering an individual to feel balanced and strong within his or her own body, yoga enhances resilience. Through these practices many young people develop the capacity to reflect before acting, limiting impulsivity. Yoga promotes cooperation and creative thinking, improving learning readiness.

Yoga is self-rewarding in many ways: Most postures get easier with practice; the poses and breathing help many students feel more relaxed after just a few moments. The lessons provide teachers with tools for modeling compassionate interaction among students. Doing yoga makes the teacher feel better, too, and this spills over into the classroom experience for all.

Response to Crisis

Sadly, many school yoga programs have been introduced as a result of national or school-wide crises. Bent on Learning was implemented in New York City after the devastation of September 11, 2001. The Lineage Project of New York City traces back to 1999, in an effort to reach disenfranchised youth who were incarcerated at Rikers Island, the city's largest jail. Yoga in Schools was implemented in a Pittsburgh elementary school plagued with high crime, high poverty levels, and high levels of incarceration among family members. Several San Francisco middle schools introduced the Quiet Time meditation program to help children cope with extreme violence in the schools and surrounding community (Fears, 2014).

After the suicide of a Portland, Oregon, student in 2013, the Wilson High School principal added Peace in Schools, a yoga and mindfulness program, as a for-credit course (House, 2014). Because of high levels of social and scholastic pressure, Newton, Massachusetts, middle schools implemented yoga, meditation, and breathing practices in their classrooms in 2012. After three teens took their lives during the 2014 school year, the district engaged the Benson Henry Institute of Mind-Body Medicine, based at Massachusetts General Hospital, in an effort to support stressed-out students, parents, and educators (Zimmerman, 2014).

Many of today's youth are in crisis. According to a Children's Defense Fund (2010) report, suicide is the third leading cause of death among 15–24-year-olds. In fact, one of every four high school students has experienced depressive symptoms severe enough to negatively impact their daily lives. The American Psychological Association (2014) reports that teens are experiencing health-threatening stress levels. Peaking during the school year, high stress negatively impacts school performance and social interactions. Due to inactivity and poor diet, obesity is rampant—affecting nearly one of every five children over age 5 in 2010 (National Center for Health Statistics, 2012).

Yoga: A Curriculum for Calm

Yoga is a movement therapy that has been proven to mitigate symptoms of stress. An excellent tool for meeting children wherever they are, it encompasses every modality of learning—visual, auditory, kinesthetic, and tactile. There are opportunities to listen, share, move, play, interact, and be still. Yoga promotes good health, self-awareness, self-esteem, and self-regulation—the ability to self-calm. It teaches children to understand their bodies, to experience their feelings, and to embody such vague and frequently invoked concepts as relaxation and focus.

Instruction is not dependent on cognitive ability or language skill. Classes can be quiet or noisy, meditative or playful, gentle or challenging. Practice may include a full range of yoga positions or be performed while seated at a desk. Lessons can be tailored for large or small groups or for individual instruction. The sessions may last for the duration of a full class period or take just a minute or two. Noncompetitive and inclusive, yoga creates an experience of community among children of diverse skills and interests.

Once introduced to the techniques, children can learn to generalize them for use in other settings. I have observed students of all abilities implementing simple yoga breaks such as shoulder shrugs or wrist stretches during writing assignments or exams. Teachers frequently report seeing students, many of whom are high achievers, using calming breaths or shoulder circles independently to relieve stress during or in between high-stakes tests. My work with children with autism spectrum disorder (ASD) resulted in fewer outbursts during the school day (Goldberg, 2004a).

Harvard researcher Sat Bir Khalsa has studied the efficacy of yoga in public schools for over a decade:

> I think yoga is an excellent behavioral practice for the management of stress in children of all ages. Even short practices can be highly effective. They not only reduce stress significantly over the short term, they are learned as lifelong skills by those who then apply them on their own in school and at home. In fact, there are a number of established yoga and mindfulness/meditation-based in-school interventions which rely upon such brief interventions in the school day. (personal communication, January 23, 2015)

Yoga education is a fit in schools in numerous ways. It can be used for physical or health education, or as a special or elective course. Brief yoga breaks can be implemented in academic classes or used as transitions between activities. School occupational therapists and mental health counselors often incorporate aspects of yoga into their therapeutic plans. Yoga can augment social and emotional learning and mindfulness training. It works equally well for school-wide and small-group Response to Intervention or Positive Behavioral Interventions and Supports. There are yoga programs designed for the general school population, while others address exceptional needs such as autism, sensory integration, and attention-deficit/hyperactivity disorder (ADHD).

Some curricula place greater emphasis on ethical practices such as compassion and kindness, bullying prevention, and other aspects of social and emotional learning. Some programs focus primarily on physical exercise, while others work more with breathing, mindful awareness, or meditation. Some employ visual cue cards, videos, or audio recordings; others use yoga mats and props. Some classes are held in gyms or classrooms with desks pushed aside; others are designed for the classroom as it is.

There are programs that bring in outside yoga educators to lead the classes or teaching materials to facilitate instruction. A growing number of school yoga programs offer in-depth training for educators. These may be conducted at school through professional development and/or mentoring programs. Many teachers attend training outside school at independent yoga centers. Tailored to address the ages and needs of their students, programs may be daylong, weekend, or residential.

Although school yoga programs vary greatly, they generally share the following components: movement (postures), breathing exercises, relaxation techniques, mindful practices, and meditation. The yoga breaks provided in this book include each of these elements. Units are arranged by theme, with lessons consisting of 1- to 5-minute exercises for use in academic classrooms. Rationale for implementation of the program includes research summaries, input from educators and yoga trainers, and over 30 years of personal experience teaching English, remedial reading, and yoga to students pre-K through college.

What Yoga Is Not

Yoga is not a religion (Feuerstein, 1998; Hyde, 2012).

Some individuals make the assumption that yoga is synonymous with Hinduism. This is incorrect. Psychologist Laura Douglass asserts, "To think Hinduism is about stretching the body, breathing practices, or even meditation is to greatly misunderstand the complexity and depth of the Hindu religion" (2010, p. 165).

One of my favorite adult students was born in India and has been a practicing Hindu all of her life. She immigrated to the United States as a young bride. Now a grandmother, it was when she moved to Florida four years ago that she was introduced to yoga and meditation. It has helped her a great deal with a number of health issues. She remains a steadfast student of yoga and Hinduism—each separate and important in her life (personal communication, November 2, 2015).

In 2014, a court case was brought by two families who objected to yoga as part of their children's elementary school's physical education program in Encinitas, California, on religious grounds. Their suit against the schools was dismissed in Superior Court and the dismissal upheld by the Fourth District Court of Appeal in April 2015. The panel of judges wrote that yoga "cannot be said to be *inherently* religious or overtly sectarian" (Court of Appeal, 2015, p. 30). In its final statement, the court found the school yoga program to be "devoid of any religious, mystical or spiritual trappings" (p. 36).

Dr. Geoff McKee is a high school principal in south Florida. The yoga program in his school, Move Through Yoga, is offered for either physical education or elective credit and is taught by educators who are also yoga teachers. It has been extremely well received among a wide array of students—from athletes hoping to improve stamina to young people who are struggling with low self-esteem. I had the opportunity to ask him if he had encountered resistance from parents or students about including the yoga program in his school. Dr. McKee responded,

> We have students from 75 countries, representing every major religious and cultural set of beliefs. From the students, parents, and teachers who are familiar with [the school yoga program], I have not heard of any offense taken in response to any element of the curriculum. As a conservative Christian, principal, and parent of an enrolled student, I have found Move Through Yoga to be complementary to the spiritual, physical, and mental wellness I seek for my children, my staff, and myself. (personal communication, February 2, 2015)

Research Update

Based on a systematic review, research on yoga for youth, although limited, suggests an array of benefits: "Yoga may be an option for children to increase physical activity and fitness. In particular, yoga may be a gateway for adopting a healthy, active lifestyle for sedentary children who are intimidated by more vigorous forms of exercise" (Birdee et al., 2009, p. 217). This review also acknowledged potential benefits for children with symptoms of ADHD.

The National Health Statistics Report of the Centers for Disease Control specified that yoga for school-aged children has been used increasingly in the United States to address pain, anxiety, and symptoms of ADHD (Black et al.,

2015). Yoga is recognized as a complementary health approach for youth by the National Institutes of Health. The report suggests that the low cost and ease of practicing yoga may contribute to its growing use and popularity among youth (Abcarian, 2013; Black et al., 2015).

Yoga for schools is a relatively new field of study. Harvard researcher Sat Bir Khalsa has determined that fewer than 50 trials on yoga in schools have been published in peer-reviewed journals (Khalsa & Butzer, 2016).

In 2012, Serwacki and Cook-Cottone reviewed 12 published studies of school yoga programs. Among the reported outcomes were lower stress levels and pulse rates for children with ASD (Goldberg, 2004a) and increased self-confidence and participation in class for children with emotional and behavioral difficulties (Powell et al., 2008). Yoga interventions resulted in fewer incidents of intrusive thoughts and impulsivity in inner city students (Mendelson et al., 2010) and less body dissatisfaction among those with eating disorder behaviors (Scime & Cook-Cottone, 2008).

School yoga has also been correlated with increased self-regulation skills and easier transitions between activities within the school day (Yoga Calm, 2007), reduced school referrals (Mindful Practices, 2015), improved self-control (Parker et al., 2014), lower levels of hostility (Frank et al., 2014), better anger control (Khalsa et al., 2012), increased time on task (Peck et al., 2005), and improved behavior and academic performance (Slovacek et al., 2003).

School Yoga Movement

The school yoga movement is growing rapidly. In 2015, Harvard researchers conducted an informal survey of 36 U.S. school yoga training programs geared toward the general education population. With nearly 5,400 yoga instructors, their combined reach is 940 schools across the country (Butzer, Ebert, et al., 2015). Yoga Ed., for example, is in 42 states and 16 countries (see http://yogaed .com/about/about-us/). Yoga 4 Classrooms estimates over 100,000 students reached (personal communication, July 12, 2015), and Yoga Calm has trained over 6,000 teachers, counselors, and therapists (see http://www.yogacalm .org/). YogaKids Tools for Schools, which has been in existence for 21 years, has 120 trained instructors, and Little Flower Yoga's School Yoga Project serves 24 schools in the New York City area (Butzer, Ebert, et al., 2015).

Creative Relaxation, my own program, has been offering direct instruction and in-service training in public schools since 1982. The target audience has been children with autism and exceptional needs, although many teachers integrate the techniques into their general education classrooms. Since the certification program was established in 2010, over 100 educators have completed the Level 2 training program (see http://www.yogaforspecialneeds.com). Countless others have implemented the program from introductory training and using my book, *Yoga Therapy for Children with Autism and Special Needs* (Goldberg, 2013) and DVD, *Creative Relaxation: Yoga for Children* (Goldberg, 2004b).

I suspect that there are many other yoga educators who, like me, have been teaching mind-body techniques in their local classrooms for many years without tracking the dozens or hundreds or thousands of children we've reached. I have spoken with many educators who, after discovering the benefits of yoga for themselves, introduced it in their own classrooms or schools. Even without formal training, they have found it rewarding for their students.

Karma Lynn Carpenter is founder of the International Association for School Yoga and Mindfulness (K-12YOGA.org). The web-based project has surveyed over 120 school-based health programs worldwide, and provides information and technical support for program implementation. Carpenter estimates that well over 50,000 teachers use mind-body tools in their classrooms today, with or without support and training. "Mindful movement potentiates the learning process. Yoga teaches children to use their brains in a way that includes their body, bridging the body and mind" (Carpenter, personal communication, April 26, 2016).

As the school yoga movement grows, annual forums such as Kripalu's Yoga in Schools Symposium and the National Kids Yoga Conference, both of which began in 2014, provide opportunities for school yoga educators to meet and exchange research data, experiences, and tools for serving youth. Published in 2015, *Best Practices for Yoga in Schools* (Childress & Cohen Harper) is a collaborative effort among school yoga educators to address challenges and offer guidelines for the implementation of yoga in classrooms. Bethany Butzer and Lisa Flynn (2016) have compiled a *Research Repository*, available online and updated quarterly. This free resource lists peer-reviewed research articles on yoga, meditation, and mindfulness for youth in schools.

PART II

MEETING SCHOOL NEEDS

School yoga "launches [a] whole-mind, brain-body educational system. The body moves into the poses, and the brain creates neural pathways and increases its learning potential. A pose may help teach math, ecology, anatomy, music, and more. The poses are the stepping stones to all of the other elements [of yoga], which creates even more avenues to learning" (Wenig, 2003, p. 10).

CHAPTER 3

Yoga as a Complement to Mindfulness Training

B EING MINDFUL MEANS being immersed in the experience of the moment, rather than anticipating what may be coming next or anguishing about what has been. Mindfulness is the practice of paying close attention, without judgment or commentary. Mindful awareness can be applied to varied activities—exercising, studying, a leisurely walk, quiet sitting, or even rushing to class. It's a system for living in the now.

Origins of Mindfulness

Like yoga, mindfulness has ancient roots. It is believed to have originated with the teachings of Siddhartha, who lived approximately 2,400 years ago (Norman, 1997). *Foundations of Mindfulness*, from the Buddhist tradition, includes awareness in four areas: the body, the feelings, the mind, and mental qualities.

- Mindfulness of the body comes by observing the posture and breathing.

- Mindfulness of the feelings comes by paying attention to physical and mental sensations.
- Mindfulness of the mind comes through awareness of thoughts.
- Mindfulness of mental qualities includes noticing distractions such as anger, worry, and desire (Jotika & Dhamminda, 1986).

Mindfulness in this ancient tradition includes an aspect of detachment: identifying posture and breathing patterns without judging them; identifying a thought or feeling without letting it define you—"not I, not mine, not self, but just a phenomenon" (Jotika & Dhamminda, 1986, p. 20). To redirect a scattered mind, *Foundations of Mindfulness* offers these strategies: body scanning, mindful breathing, and the practice of loving-kindness (Jotika & Dhamminda, 1986). Each of these is also an essential aspect of yoga breaks for classrooms.

Body scanning, concentrating on specific areas of the body, is a technique used to develop "one-pointedness" in yoga. This is the ability to attend to one thing at one time, without judgment, using the body as a focal point (see Unit 2, Floating on a Cloud; and Unit 4, Focusing Practice).

Breath awareness, one of the foundational rungs of the yoga teachings, may be included in any yoga posture. The BREATHE FIRST curriculum includes an introductory unit dedicated to instruction in breathing—in stillness and movement (see Unit 1). Each subsequent unit of the curriculum includes lessons for observing the breath.

The practice of kindness is one of the tenets of yoga. The concept of avoiding harm—to oneself and others—sets the tone for all instruction (see Chapter 1 and Guidelines for Classroom Yoga Breaks in Chapter 14).

Mindfulness Today

Institutions of higher learning have been instrumental in bringing mindfulness education into the mainstream. Naropa University in Boulder, Colorado, was founded in 1974 by a renowned Tibetan Buddhist. "His vision was to take the very best elements of western scholarship and combine them with an emphasis on eastern wisdom tradition" (Naropa University, 2015). Contemplative education with rigorous academics and community engagement is their model for undergraduate and graduate studies.

A secular form of mindfulness has become highly regarded in the science and practice of well-being, according to the University of California Greater Good Science Center (2015). Launched in 1979 at the University of Massachusetts Medical School, Jon Kabat-Zinn's Mindfulness-Based Stress Reduction (MBSR) program has helped move mindfulness practices into mainstream America. "Since that time, thousands of studies have documented the physical and mental health benefits of mindfulness in general and MBSR in particular, inspiring countless programs to adapt the MBSR model for schools, prisons, hospitals, veterans centers, and beyond" (Greater Good Science Center, 2015).

Kabat-Zinn defines mindfulness as "paying attention in a particular way: on purpose, in the present moment, and nonjudgmentally" (1994, p. 4). He describes MBSR as an educational (rather than therapeutic) system for reducing stress and building community support; qualities such as patience, acceptance, and letting go are key elements (Kabat-Zinn, 1996).

MBSR includes a number of practices in common with yoga: breathing exercises, gentle yoga postures, sitting meditation, and body scanning. Both yoga and MBSR emphasize kindness and connecting with community.

In her book *Mindfulness for Teachers*, Patricia Jennings describes different forms of mindful awareness practice. Whereas seated meditation and slow mindful movement are formal practices, mindfulness may also be practiced informally, during routine activities throughout the day: "At any given moment you can bring mindful awareness to . . . external sounds, objects, other people or animals, and internal thoughts, sensations, and feelings" (Jennings, 2015, p. 3).

There is a distinction between mindfulness and relaxation, according to Learning to Breathe (L2B) author Patricia Broderick. Paying attention to and feeling our emotions may not be relaxing; these are, however, important aspects of being fully present (personal communication, April 27, 2015).

Mindfulness for Schools

Mindfulness has shown promise as an intervention. Studies have shown benefits for students with symptoms of ADHD (Zylowska et al., 2008; Van de Weijer-Bergsma et al., 2012), in lowering levels of anxiety and depression (Biegel et al., 2009), better academic performance (Beauchemin et al., 2008), improvements in self-regulation (Broderick & Metz, 2009), decreased aggression (Schonert-Reichl & Lawlor, 2010), lowered depressive symptoms in minority children (Liehr & Diaz, 2010), and enhanced overall well-being (Huppert & Johnson, 2010).

According to a systematic review and meta-analysis of mindfulness programs for schools, "Mindfulness practice enhances the very qualities and goals of education in the 21st century . . . includ[ing] . . . attentional and emotional self-regulation, . . . prosocial dispositions such as empathy and compassion, . . . ethical sensitivity, creativity, and problem solving skills" (Zenner et al., 2014, p. 2).

The school mindfulness programs examined in the meta-analysis were diverse. One constant, however, was breathing practices, which were included in 100% of the programs reviewed. Over half of the programs used body scans, and almost as many included body practices like yoga or mindful movement. Other common elements were working with thoughts and feelings, awareness of sensations, and kindness practices (Zenner et al., 2014).

Classroom implementation of school mindfulness programs may vary in duration from brief pauses interjected by classroom teachers to extended school-wide curricula. The diverse programs include "contemplative approaches such as yoga, tai chi, and relaxation which may be more likely to appeal to energetic youth than sitting meditation alone" (Weare, 2015, p. 255). Patricia Jennings agrees that practices that involve body awareness are especially appropriate for youth (personal communication, May 15, 2015). In a study that examined mindfulness relative to executive function in elementary school children, movement was an important element in each session (Flook et al., 2010).

Mindfulness training is also available for educators. Cultivating Awareness and Resilience in Education for Teachers, offered by the Garrison Institute, teaches mindfulness and self-regulation practices that have been shown to improve personal well-being and classroom management skills (Jennings et al., 2012).

Yoga and Mindfulness

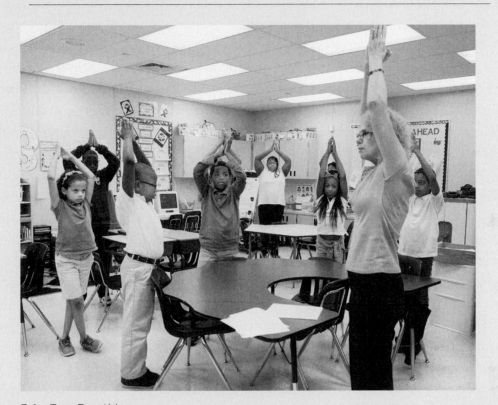

3-1   Tree Breathing

Yoga is a practice of mindful movement, directing awareness to the body, breath, and feelings in every pose. Students learn to observe their bodies—how it feels when they are in motion, when they are still, when they breathe in and out. They learn to observe their minds—whether they are distracted, anxious, or calm. By learning to identify these feelings, without judging them, young people discover the distinction between agitation that comes from outside and that which comes from within. Learning that they can control their inner responses is the first step in managing stress.

A moving meditation, yoga creates opportunities to experience a deeper sense of self. In addition, yoga builds nonjudgmental connections with others by creating inclusive communities.

Harvard Medical School neuroscientist Sat Bir Khalsa believes that "yoga is a mindfulness practice. It promotes fitness, but it is much more than exercise. Yoga reduces stress and teaches kids to focus attention, thereby increasing attention skills and mind-body awareness" (personal communication, February 19, 2015). Research supports that contention. A 2009 study explored the impact of an 8-week yoga intervention on mindfulness. The results, using the Freiburg Mindfulness Inventory, "indicate that the yoga group experienced a significant increase in overall mindfulness, and in three mindfulness subscales: Attention to the present moment, Accepting and open attitudes toward experience, and Insightful understanding" (Shelov et al., 2009, p. 595).

Sitting still is challenging for many young people. Yet it's how they spend most of their school days. School counselor Beth Johnson is a yoga teacher and MindUp workshop facilitator. When teaching mindfulness at the elementary school level, she found that "Yoga is a perfect way for children to experience mindful movement. After even a minute or two practicing yoga poses, students were able to refocus their attention and move forward with the task at hand" (personal communication, July 2, 2016).

Programs that combine rhythmic movement and breathing exercises make meditation practices more accessible for individuals of varying abilities (Shannahoff-Khalsa, 2010). A study examining the practice of meditation for children on the autism spectrum suggests a variety of techniques, including the use of rhythm, chant, and movement. "Successful programs do not require that children remain sitting still for very long but encourage social bonding, joy, and confidence" (Sequeira & Ahmed, 2012, p. 6).

According to the National Health Statistics Report of the Centers for Disease Control, most children practiced "traditional forms of yoga . . . not simply yoga as exercise," which included meditation and deep breathing exercises. In fact, meditation was included as part of movement therapies—either yoga, tai chi, or qigong—among 80% of the more than 90,000 children who used meditation in 2012 (Black et al., 2015, p. 7).

Yoga cultivates the faculties of concentration and one-pointedness. The objective in yoga is not how much or how fast you can do; rather, it's how aware you can be in the doing; how still in the not-doing. The physical body—whether in motion or at rest—provides a focal point. Students develop the ability to scan their bodies for tension and release unneeded holding from their muscles. By noticing the ease as well as the resistance in a posture, children learn to accept, understand, and simply be in their own bodies.

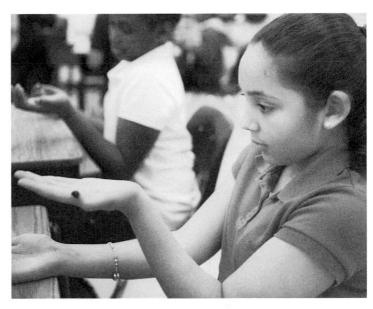

3-2   Palm Gazing

With practice, many students learn the process of watching the mind without judging, even as it hops from thought to thought. They may start by simply observing the inhalation and exhalation or focusing on the palm of their hand. In postures, they begin redirecting their awareness to the breath while in motion. With consistent practice in yoga class, many find that breath awareness spills over into other activities—while taking tests, competing in sports, or during difficult social interactions. Using their breath as an anchor, students discover the power of a focused mind, one that is under the control of its owner.

Two Sides of a Cloth: Body and Mind

It is certainly possible to practice mindfulness without doing yoga, as evidenced by the varied approaches to this vast subject. The practice of yoga, however, must be performed mindfully. Focused attention, without judgment, is what distinguishes yoga from other forms of exercise.

Yoga master B. K. S. Iyengar explains the role of mindfulness in yoga: "The mind is the vital link between the body and the consciousness. The individual can live with awareness, discrimination, and confidence only once the mind is calm and focused. Yoga . . . generates this equilibrium" (2001, p. 26). My teacher Swami Vishnudevananda frequently stated, "You can't wash one side of a cloth."

Mind and body, like the front and back of a piece of cloth, are inseparable. You may see only one side, but you can't alter one without influencing the other. By making the body more limber, you open the doorways within the mind. By strengthening the physical body, you strengthen your resolve. By focusing on the breath, you deepen the capacity to attend.

It takes just a moment to interject a mindful yoga break within the school day, as you'll see in the BREATHE FIRST curriculum. By breathing, standing, sitting, and moving with awareness, students learn to become astute observers of their bodies and minds. These features of yoga are consistent with the tenets of mindfulness.

CHAPTER 4

Yoga as a Complement to Social and Emotional Learning

COLLABORATIVE FOR ACADEMIC, Social, and Emotional Learning (CASEL), founded in 1994, is an organization dedicated to promoting the inclusion of evidence-based social and emotional learning (SEL) strategies for students at all grade levels. CASEL defines SEL as a process for acquiring tools for managing emotions, setting and achieving goals, increasing empathy and positive relationships, and making responsible choices. SEL strategies are based on the importance of supportive relationships to "make learning challenging, engaging, and meaningful" (CASEL, 2015).

In addition to promoting skills in the five competencies discussed below, SEL programs have been instrumental in "creating positive learning environments that are safe, caring, engaging, and participatory, and improving student attitudes and beliefs about self, others, and school" (CASEL, 2015). Research demonstrates that SEL has improved social interactions among classmates and throughout the school environment; decreased conduct disruptions, aggressive acts, and referrals; lessened student stress levels and incidence of depression;

increased motivation and commitment to learning; and improved academic performance by approximately 11% (Durlak et al., 2011; Greenberg et al., 2003).

The five competencies for SEL are

- Self-awareness
- Self-management
- Social awareness
- Relationship skills
- Responsible decision making (CASEL, 2015)

While yoga is not a substitute for SEL, it is well suited to support the competencies of SEL. The yoga breaks described in this book are rooted in Creative Relaxation, the therapeutic yoga intervention that I developed and have been implementing in schools since 1982. Its principles parallel many of those within the guidelines for SEL. As you'll see over the following pages, yoga breaks within the school day offer a peaceful space for young people to reflect and reconnect with their center. By providing opportunities to have fun and engage with classmates—without judgment or competition—yoga helps build empathy and a sense of community. Students learn healthy tools to relieve frustration, improve focus, and self-regulate, enhancing academic and social success. Yoga fosters resilience and independence, supporting better decision making.

Let's examine specific ways that yoga complements the SEL competencies.

- Self-awareness: The ability to accurately recognize one's emotions and thoughts and their influence on behavior. This includes accurately assessing one's strengths and limitations and possessing a well-grounded sense of confidence and optimism (CASEL, 2015).

Young people, especially adolescents, are highly influenced by the world that surrounds them—friends, fashion, star power, sex appeal. Their preoccupation with what others think can be all-consuming. This external focus, however, is not helpful in learning to manage their own behaviors and thinking. As psychiatrist Bessel van der Kolk noted from his work with individuals recovering from PTSD, research demonstrates that the best method to manage one's own feelings is by first becoming aware of the "*inner* experience, and accepting what they find" (2014, p. 206).

Yoga is a practice of self-awareness. Quietly observing the body while in motion and in stillness, students learn to notice the feeling, rhythm, and depth of their breathing. In yoga postures, they are guided to pay attention to the position of each hand and foot, their head, and where to fix their gaze. This process of mindful focus in yoga can also become a tool for behavior management. Students learn where they are holding tension, how it makes them feel, and techniques for its release.

As Dan Siegel points out in *Brainstorm*, it is during adolescence that the "ability to reflect on our personalities emerges" (2013, p. 90). While some of this is genetically determined, experience also plays a role: "What we focus our attention on and what we spend time doing directly stimulates the growth of the parts of the brain that carry out those functions" (p. 90).

Becoming students of their own bodies and minds, as practiced in yoga, young people develop patterns of awareness that overlap into other areas of their life.

- Self-management: The ability to regulate one's emotions, thoughts, and behaviors effectively in different situations. This includes managing stress, controlling impulses, motivating oneself, and setting and working toward achieving personal and academic goals (CASEL, 2015).

Allison Morgan, founder of Zensational Kids, asks, "What makes kids behave the way they do? It's how they feel. If we help them become aware of how they feel, then they can recognize that there are things they can do to change those feelings."

For dealing with anger, Morgan suggests Lion pose, also called Dragon Breath, where the breath is released in a roar. "I explain to them that when you are angry, it's like having a ball of fire in your belly. It almost hurts. You might push or yell or hurt someone else without meaning to, just to try to get the fire out, but it's not going to work. But if you remember to breathe like a dragon and release that fire from your belly, you will feel better much more quickly and so will everyone else around you" (personal communication, April 15, 2016).

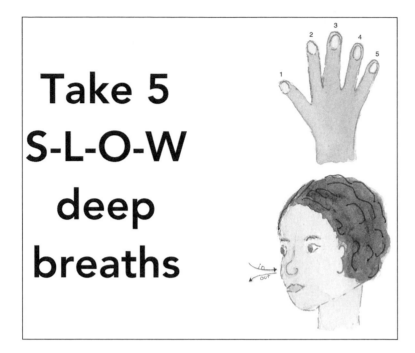

4-1   "Take 5" S.T.O.P.
and Relax

When developing S.T.O.P. and Relax (Goldberg, Miller, Collins, & Morales, 2006), a visual yoga-based curriculum, my colleagues and I started with small group instruction with children in autism clusters. To help with self-management, we designed illustrated cue cards with calming techniques that children practiced regularly in the relaxation sessions. Attached to students' schedules and sometimes fixed right on their desks, the cards served as reminders to take five slow breaths or open their chests at designated intervals throughout their day (Goldberg et al., 2006).

Some of these students also spent a portion of their day in general education classes. To reinforce these skills, we shared the same relaxation techniques with their entire class. By providing self-regulation skills to all of the students, the classroom teacher and the student community supported implementation of these methods as needed. Teachers reported seeing children cueing their classmates to "take 5" when they seemed on the verge of an upset. Many in the general class population also reported using these self-calming techniques to manage their own stress during school testing and interactions with others (Collins & Goldberg, 2012). You will find examples of yoga breaks to enhance self-management skills in Parts IV and V.

• Social awareness: The ability to take the perspective of and empathize with others from diverse backgrounds and cultures, to understand social and ethical norms for behavior, and to recognize family, school, and community resources and supports.

In addition to my work as a consultant and trainer for educators, I teach weekly children's yoga classes. The community within my classes is diverse. Boys and girls range in age from 5 to 18 years old; children with exceptional challenges are integrated with children from general education classes. One of the most compelling experiences for me is watching children adapt to others who are very different—in size, strength, flexibility, and general capacity. There are opportunities for children to assist one another, to learn patience and compassion, and to make new friends.

Many of the students that I work with have exceptional needs, including autism, ADHD, and sensory processing disorder. Fitting in can be challenging for these students. Some have difficulty negotiating personal boundaries—how close is too close? How far is standoffish? Others may not recognize the impact of their words on others—that telling the unfiltered truth can be hurtful and may not always be necessary. Some children do not realize that other people have different ways of understanding and assessing life's experiences. This can make it very difficult for them to see someone else's point of view or to recognize how their own behaviors may be viewed by others.

There is research showing that imitation, a skill that many individuals with ASD do not inherently possess, is an antecedent to empathy (Iacoboni, 2008) and that the more empathetic an individual is, the better his or her social skills (Medina, 2012). Much of yoga instruction is demonstration, and its practice is imitation. Because yoga is noncompetitive and adaptive, there are many different ways of performing postures. This provides teachers an extraordinary opportunity to model appropriate forms of interaction among individuals of varied skills and learning styles.

Yoga has been shown to improve imitation skills, eye contact, and interactive play among children with ASD (Radhakrishna, 2010). Rhythmic movements and breathing practices have increased focus and imitation skills for children on the autism spectrum (Shannahoff-Khalsa, 2010). These are important social skills for all students.

Brynne Caleda of Yoga Ed. comments on yoga for social awareness for students and teachers:

> Internal changes in oneself naturally lead to external changes in our interactions with others. Class discussion, partner postures, and group activities are opportunities for students to share their own experiences and understand their classmates' experiences.
>
> The Yoga Ed. teaching philosophy also encourages educators to be more socially aware of their students' backgrounds, behaviors, and needs. . . . Empathy allows you to experience what your students are experiencing. These techniques promote your social awareness and allow you to [more] effectively teach. (personal communication, April 1, 2014)

In yoga, students practice techniques to change not only how they feel about themselves, but how others perceive them. Learning to stand their ground in Warrior poses is an excellent example. Even a child who feels insecure in the presence of others can learn to project confidence in this posture. Standing with his weight evenly distributed on both feet, with the back aligned and arms upright, the child embodies strength and power, rather than presenting himself as a potential victim.

You'll find more techniques for setting the tone within your classroom, as well as examples of the role of yoga in community building and teaching empathy, in chapter 15.

- Relationship skills: The ability to establish and maintain healthy and rewarding relationships with diverse individuals and groups. This includes communicating clearly, listening actively, cooperating, resisting inappropriate social pressure, negotiating conflict constructively, and seeking and offering help when needed.

Within a yoga lesson, there are ways for children of diverse talents and strengths to connect and serve one another. One of the most effective techniques I have employed in school yoga is inviting children from general education classes to serve as models and guides for classmates with exceptional needs or to select students from upper grades to assist those in lower grades. Both the helper and

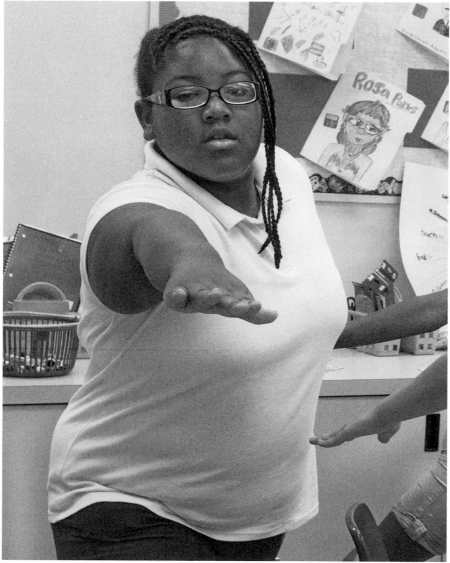

4-2   Focused Warrior 2

the learner develop skills in acceptance, listening, and effective communication (Goldberg, 2013). Many of the yoga educators whom I spoke with shared stories of unlikely friendships and bonds formed among their students.

Partner yoga is an excellent tool for learning that how you treat others matters. Students deal with the natural consequences of their behavior with their classmates. When holding hands in Flying Bats, for example, if one lets go before

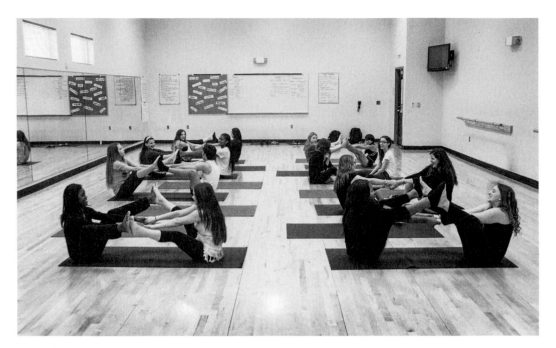

4-3   Flying Bats

the other, the partner will fall backward. There's a lot to learn about trust in these poses.

Sometimes, what is difficult for one student becomes easier by working with others. If a student is struggling with Tree Balance, for example, he may find that practicing with a partner helps. Standing side by side, each student offers support and stability to the other. It requires negotiation and adaptation—both verbal and subtle forms of communication. At the same time, partner poses make the experience a lot of fun.

Playful banter, assisting others, and working as a team are all skills developed through the practice of yoga. Research has shown that elementary school students who participated in school yoga programs were less inclined to bully others and less likely to be victimized by their peers (Marie, Wyshak, & Wyshak, 2008). Aggressive and retaliative behaviors were also reduced among yoga participants (Frank et al., 2014). For more information on bullying, see Chapter 7.

- Responsible decision making: The ability to make constructive and respectful choices about personal behavior and social interactions

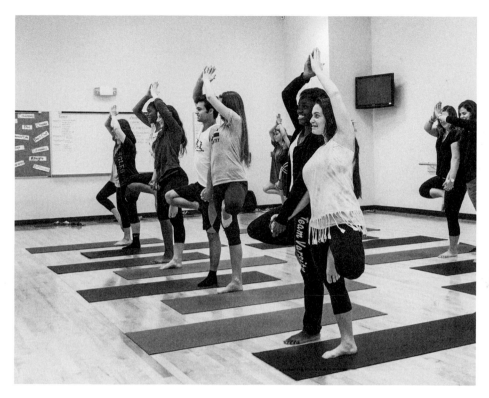

4-4   Partner Tree Balance

based on consideration of ethical standards, safety concerns, social norms, the realistic evaluation of consequences of various actions, and the well-being of self and others.

Patricia Broderick's Learning to Breathe (L2B) curriculum combines mindful awareness practices, group activities, and mindful movements. Research has found reductions in depression and anxiety levels and increases in emotion regulation among adolescents using L2B in school programs. Students said they experienced a greater sense of control in their reactions to stressors after participating in the L2B program (Broderick, personal communication, April 15, 2016).

Learning to tune in and feel the body, to notice the shifts in breathing, to observe what is going on in the gut is useful for many forms of behavior management, including decision making. Before making an important decision, for example, children can learn to check in with their body. "How does it feel in my

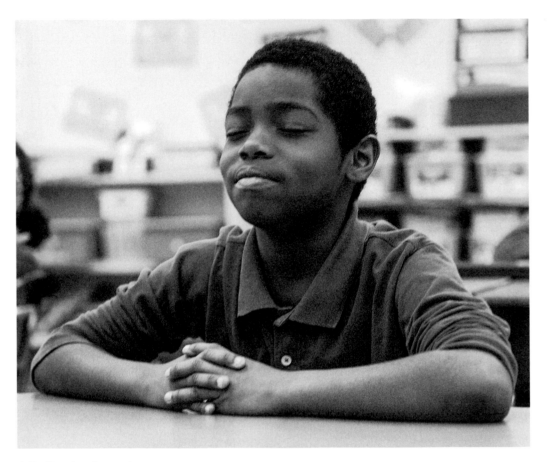

4-5   Turning Inward

chest when I join with my friends who are teasing that boy on the bus? What happens in my belly when I tell my mother a lie?"

Learning to listen to and acknowledge information that comes from the gut makes us better problem solvers. "Gut feelings are messages from the insula and other bottom-up circuits that simplify life decisions for us by guiding our attention upward to smarter options" (Goleman, 2013, p. 66). Daniel Siegel describes this as "gist thinking, when adolescents start to use judgment . . . informed by experience and intuition" rather than the drive for reward (2013, p. 83). He adds that "intuition plays a very important role in making good decisions" (p. 71).

Interestingly, research has revealed that the brains of meditators have thicker insulas than those of nonmeditators (Lazar et al., 2005). Exercise has been shown to enhance problem-solving skills (Hillman, Buck, Themanson, Pontifex, & Castelli, 2009; Hillman, Erickson, & Kramer, 2008; Hillman et al., 2006; Medina, 2008; Ratey with Hagerman, 2008), and children who practice yoga have demonstrated improved reasoning skills and executive function—the ability to assess, plan, and follow through (Diamond, 2012; Gothe et al., 2013). For more on yoga and executive function, see Chapter 13.

CHAPTER 5

Yoga as a Complement to Physical Education

YOGA IMPROVES BALANCE, strength, and flexibility through movement; increases endurance and focus through breathing techniques; and increases body-mind awareness. Its noncompetitive structure fosters community and acceptance among peers.

A noncontact exercise program, yoga is accessible to students with sensory sensitivities and diverse physical abilities. Partnering is an optional form of practice, and when used, encourages cooperation rather than competition. Even in a crowded gymnasium, yoga mats establish natural boundaries between students, clarifying personal space and facilitating class discipline.

Yoga is complementary to other fitness programs. A review of studies comparing the benefits of yoga and aerobic exercise found yoga "as effective as or better than exercise at improving a variety of health-related outcome measures" (Ross & Thomas, 2010, p. 3). Postures may be implemented as warm-ups to begin class or cool-downs after other forms of exercise (see Appendix 4 for specific warm-up and cool-down sequences). Breathing awareness is useful in varied sports and physical activities. The sense of self-control and self-awareness that students learn through yoga often enhances their capacity for better sportsmanship and team activities. By experiencing mastery over their own bodies, students may revise their body images. Improved self-regulation skills help students to postpose gratification and assess a situation before reacting. The stress management tools that students learn when yoga is combined with PE serve them in coping with athletic, academic, and social challenges.

Yoga is becoming an essential part of many athletic training programs. Chris Theodore, founder of Theoga, is a PE teacher who incorporates yoga in his curriculum in the Philadelphia school district. He says, "Serious athletes need to be challenged, so I teach tough balance poses. Then, depending on their response, I can make it harder or easier—whatever it takes to keep their interest." Theodore notes that student athletes are under a lot of pressure. "I coach the guys on the crew team to focus on their breath. It keeps them centered. When a basketball player is standing on the foul line to take an important shot, he can learn to use his breathing to shut out the noise of the crowd" (personal communication, August 9, 2014).

Coaches from Melrose High in St. Cloud, Minnesota, have added yoga for flexibility and focus training to their sports teams' regimen. One of the football coaches explains that through yoga, "We're trying to get them to relax, breathe and stretch." The girls' swim team has also added yoga after competitions. In addition to core strength and stretching, the emphasis in yoga is on "staying centered" (Rennecke, 2015).

Pittsburgh public school PE teachers who implemented the Yoga in Schools program reported improved classroom management, particularly when yoga routines were practiced at the beginning of class. They also observed more time on task and greater inclusion among nonathletic youth. Both teachers and pupils appreciated the calming effects of yoga in their PE classes (Spence, 2014).

Student athletes may be inspired to know that many professional athletes find yoga helpful for their game. In June 2014, *Sports Illustrated* featured a story about the use of yoga among National Basketball Association (NBA) players, with photos of LeBron James, Kevin Love, and Dirk Nowitzki in varied yoga postures. Los Angeles Clippers' star Blake Griffin explained, "I think it's huge for guys to start young and realize the benefits [of yoga]. . . . When you take care of your body through yoga, it extends years on your career. I do think it will become more and more the norm in the NBA" (Toland, 2014).

National Football League (NFL) teams such as the Philadelphia Eagles and Seattle Seahawks also practice yoga on a regular basis. Professional football player Jeremy Cain has played for teams including the Chicago Bears, Tennessee Titans, and Jacksonville Jaguars during his 12-year career in the NFL. A 2011 injury resulting in an intensely painful herniated disc and nerve damage led him to yoga with Joy Elsner:

> She researched long snappers (my position) to understand the movement and skill required while playing. After a few beginner classes, she taught me specific yoga postures that would strengthen me on the field.
>
> After I was healed and my nerves regenerated, I noticed a significant difference: I had increased my core strength and overall balance, which translated well for my role on the field. The most surprising part about yoga is how well it improved my focus. When I'm in a yoga pose, I don't think about anything except keeping my body strong and balanced.
>
> Yoga instruction is much more than physical postures—it has helped me be in the moment by breathing and relaxing my mind. Then I'm able to center myself and consistently execute under pressure. There is so much adversity, so many ups and downs in football. Yoga has taught me to be present minded. (Jeremy Cain, personal communication, February 3, 2015)

See Appendix 5 for Jeremy Cain's personal centering, strength, and balance routine.

University of Texas clinical professor Dolly Lambdin believes that including yoga is "one sign of a high-quality PE program" (Roth, 2014). Lambdin, past president of SHAPE America, the Society of Health and Physical Educators, affirmed, "I believe we must empower students to take ownership of their own health. Introducing students to a wide range of physical activities makes it more likely they will find an activity that they enjoy and want to pursue on a regular basis. Yoga strengthens mind-body connections and awareness and so is valuable both in physical education and in the classroom" (personal communication, December 6, 2015).

Many yoga programs align with national or local PE standards. In addition, many yoga training tools are available for including brief yoga routines within existing PE programs. Physical education teachers have used visual cue cards and posters to establish exercise stations around the gymnasium or classroom for independent practice. Yoga DVDs, available through many programs, also facilitate the implementation of yoga into PE programs.

Competition and Cooperation

Most sports are competitive by nature. It's impossible to determine a winner without a loser. Friendly competition is a positive experience—and very much a part of the American culture. Competition offers important interpersonal lessons about teamwork and sportsmanship. There's great value in learning to handle defeat as well as victory.

Competition can be highly motivating for children. It underlies their drive to succeed in school as well as athletics. The emphasis on competition, however, can also be harmful. Overemphasis on winning—often generated by parents—can make sports stressful and anxiety provoking for youths (Merkel, 2013). The pressure to win creates a fear of failure among some children; for some, losing becomes a source of self-recrimination (Engh, 2002).

During competitive sporting events, adolescents may succumb to goading from peers, resulting in choices they later regret (Hansen et al., 2003). Pressure to perform sometimes encourages youths to disregard their bodies, playing while injured (Merkel, 2013) or exhausted. Poor athletic performance can also contribute to decreased self-confidence and loss of interest in sports (Merkel, 2013).

A study conducted in 2014 reported a significant relationship between stress, anger, and bullying in PE classes in an inner-city Detroit school (Centeio et al., 2014). There is evidence that competitive sports in PE classes foster aggressive behaviors among more dominant youths, while marginalizing less athletic youths (Ennis, 1999). Researchers from Wayne State University Department of Kinesiology suggested yoga as an alternative to competitive sports to create a less stressful environment in PE, thus reducing incidents of anger and bullying (Centeio et al., 2014). Peaceful, community-building PE programs have resulted in decreased aggressive behaviors (Ennis, 1999).

Lawn Chair is a calming posture that promotes cooperation. Students sit back to back on their mats, with legs extended. At the teacher's cue, one row

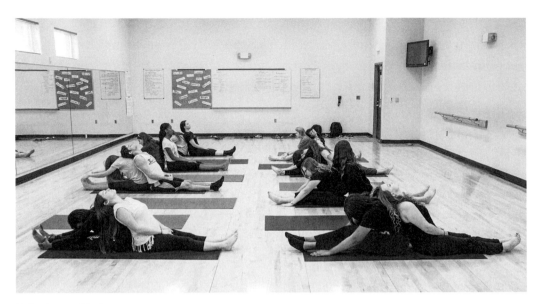

5-1   Lawn Chair

slowly folds forward while their partners rest their shoulders and head against the other's back, as if they were relaxing in a lawn chair. If students are not comfortable surrendering their heads, they may simply rest their backs on their partner. Those with tight hamstrings may prefer to bend their knees when in the forward fold position.

Together students breathe in the pose, while the teacher discusses the concept of having a teammate's back. How does it feel to support a friend in this posture, to absorb his weight? What about for the students who are leaning back—is it difficult to let go and trust that they are safe? After a short pause, reverse the positions, so that the other student now rests on his or her partner's lawn chair, supported. Ask students to consider the same questions from their new perspective.

Physical education provides an important opportunity for students of diverse academic and physical abilities to come together as a community. Yoga postures and breathing offer tools to teach concepts such as sportsmanship and collaboration within the PE curriculum.

CHAPTER 6

Response to Intervention and Positive Behavioral Interventions and Supports

RESPONSE TO INTERVENTION (RtI) is a system of research-based interventions to address student needs that are not being met within the classroom. Students whose reading or math skills are well below grade level, for example, may be served by RtI. Although many RtIs focus primarily on academics, research suggests a greater likelihood for success when both academic and behavioral challenges are addressed (Vaughn & Fuchs, 2003).

Positive Behavioral Interventions and Supports (PBIS) is a school-wide methodology for solving and preventing behavioral problems. According to the U.S. Department of Education's Office of Special Education Programs (OSEP), research shows that punishment, especially if used without positive strategies, is not effective. OSEP emphasizes the importance of "modeling . . . and reinforcing positive social behavior" and rewarding students who follow these behaviors, rather than waiting to respond to misbehavior. "The purpose of school-wide PBIS is to establish a climate in which appropriate behavior is the norm" (OSEP, 2015).

Both RtI and PBIS employ a three-tiered approach to attaining desired outcomes. Tier 1 is global, implemented for the entire school or class. Tier 2 is used for students who have not attained the desired academic or behavioral goals. Additional instruction and support are provided within smaller groups. For those children who still haven't reached the targeted goals, Tier 3 strategies are employed in even smaller groups or with individual instruction. If Tier 3 instruction is not adequate for resolving the child's academic or social difficulties, an alternative education plan is explored.

According to Karma Lynn Carpenter, a pioneer in the school yoga and mindfulness movement and founder of K–12Yoga, RtI is a civil rights issue. "Without learning readiness, students are at risk of slipping into the school-to-prison pipeline of disability status, unemployment, crime, prison, or worse." She points to growing evidence of the effectiveness of school-based yoga and mindfulness for learning-readiness and RtI, and stresses that "localized implementation support that is culturally-aligned is crucial to success and sustainability" (personal communication, April 26, 2016).

Speaking at Kripalu's Yoga in Schools Symposium in February 2015, superintendent Cynthia Zurchin shared an extraordinary story. A first grader in the Pittsburgh public schools had been suspended from five schools before coming to hers. With one sibling in jail and another who had been shot, this child was angry and frightened. Because of his inability to manage his behavior and poor school performance, he was labeled a "thought to be" special education student.

During the course of the school year, Dr. Zurchin, who was then the school principal, instituted a program of positive reinforcement and reward. In addition, she implemented a school-wide yoga program, which she called Breathing. Her goal was to transform the school environment from one of chaos to one of calm and hope. The troubled first grader responded extremely well; his behavior and schoolwork improved dramatically. In fact, he was found to be gifted (Zurchin, 2015).

Breathing is a tool that most children can learn to use for self-regulation. Carpenter believes that "schools can make it possible for every child to have that basic civil right to manage their own behavior through their breathing" (personal communication, September 2, 2015).

School social worker Kathy Flaminio, founder of 1000 Petals, and Lynea Gillen, cofounder of Yoga Calm, have adapted school yoga to RtI and PBIS systems. Using the Yoga Calm curriculum, which includes breathing, postures, mindfulness practices, and SEL, they have designed three tiers of instruction. Here's a sample of how the intervention works.

Tier 1 includes school-wide training in mindful breathing. Student leaders model breathing using a Hoberman sphere (http://www.hoberman.com/fold/Sphere/sphere.htm). This expandable dome can be stretched during inhalation and compressed during exhalation to demonstrate the expansion and contraction of the lungs during respiration.

Tier 2 offers more consistent relaxation practices, with fewer students. Here they begin addressing more specific stress-related challenges within the smaller group. The selection of postures would depend upon the skills and needs of the students. Grounding postures such as Warrior, for example, may be used to provide

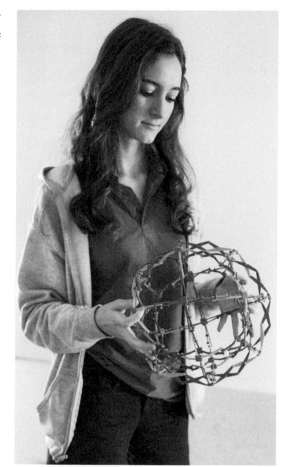

6-1   Expanded Hoberman Sphere

students a sense of stability and awareness of their connection to the earth beneath them.

Tier 3 sessions are one-on-one and meet more frequently than the other tiers. Personal routines for school or home practice are created, with postures and breathing techniques selected that best serve the needs of the individual. Tense and Relax, for example, teaches students to exaggerate and then release areas where they are holding tension (see Unit 2). In this way, they begin to learn how and where their bodies respond to stress and techniques for mitigating this response.

Kathy Flaminio shared an example of the success of this program. "One of our school administrators was asked for her suspension sheet, but she couldn't

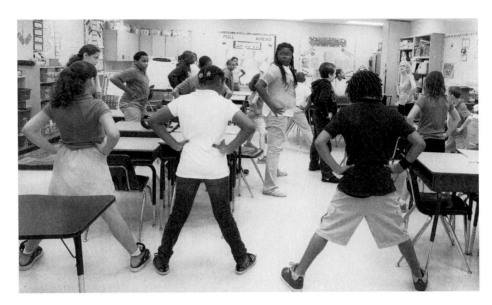

6-2   Warrior Stance

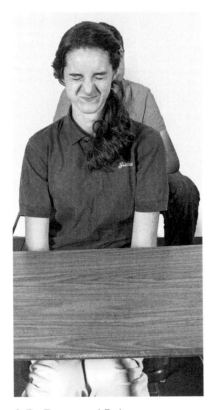

6-3   Tense and Relax

locate it. She realized that since implementing Yoga Calm and PBIS she has had no suspensions in three years!" (personal communication, September 8, 2015).

A positive, accessible intervention for self-regulation, yoga is suitable for use as an RtI or PBIS.

CHAPTER 7

Addressing Bullying Through Yoga

ADOLESCENTS TEND TO view the world as it affects and concerns them. They are often loath to consider the impact of their words and behavior on the people around them. Many of the students whom I work with seem genuinely surprised that they have done anything to contribute to another's pain, despite many obvious indications that they have. Behaviors like bullying or teasing seem innocent or inconsequential to many on the giving end, regardless of the devastation for those who receive such treatment.

School social worker Rich Foss says that one of the best deterrents to being bullied is having friends. Making connections with others and knowing that someone has your back can make all the difference in how a student feels and how he is perceived by his peers (personal communication, December 9, 2015).

Yoga, which is a noncompetitive, inclusive activity, engenders a feeling of connection. Many unlikely friendships grow from sharing yoga classes. Students frequently report being yoga buddies with kids they wouldn't ordinarily hang out with. Being from different crowds doesn't preclude being friends. One high school student with a record of fighting and expulsion explained that her yoga class felt "more like a family than a regular class." Barely holding back tears, she told me that because things were so bad at home, with so much turmoil, this meant a great deal to her. In turn, she watches out for her yoga friends, so no one from the tough crowd bothers them.

Pam Leal, a middle school yoga teacher, observes her students being inclusive of children from "exceptional education classes or those who are shy or fearful. They partner in ways that build trust and kindness" (personal communication, May 21, 2015). Countless teachers have shared stories of students who tell them that yoga is one of the only places where they feel safe and accepted.

Boundaries and Social and Emotional Learning

Working with adolescents, I see much confusion about boundaries and personal space. How close can you stand to someone without making him or her uncomfortable? For others, any encroachment into their perceived personal space is anxiety provoking. Fear sometimes leads to aggressive behavior.

These behavioral subtleties can be a challenge for young people of all abilities. Bullying may begin simply when one steps too far into another student's space. This may be something that the bully does not intend. Seeing the fear and discomfort caused by this encroachment, however, can become intoxicating. It's a power that they did not know they had, based on social mores that they may not understand.

Psychologist, author, and yoga teacher Dr. Lauren Rubenstein works with at-risk youth. She finds yoga to be an excellent tool for addressing social interaction. Rubenstein uses an exercise from *Yoga Calm* for teaching personal boundaries (Gillen & Gillen, 2008). Students form two lines facing one another on opposite sides of the room. "The active line steps forward slowly toward the passive line, one step at a time, until each one reaches the boundary of another's personal space."

After the exercise, Rubenstein asks, "'At what point did you feel uncomfortable?' It is important for both the approachers and observers to note how their own bodies signal discomfort and how to read their peers' body language. Next they practice ways to express 'that's too close' and of repositioning themselves instead of getting upset or just being polite" (personal communication, October 29, 2014).

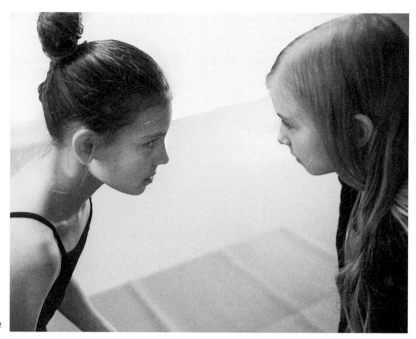

7-1 That's Too Close

Posture

Physical posture has a tremendous bearing on how a person is perceived. When a student stands erect, he sends a message of confidence. If he is feeling fearful, this may be conveyed by a slumped posture or awkward gait. A 2013 study confirmed that gait and body language were used by criminals to select the most vulnerable targets. Individuals who displayed less synchronous walks, were not paying attention, or looked fearful were more often victims of aggressive acts. On the other hand, walking with confident strides, appearing fit, and being observant resulted in being a less likely victim (Book et al., 2013).

Yoga is the science of posture. Students learn to move with awareness, to observe their feelings in a pose. There are also many positions that build strength in the large muscles of the back—the ones that help students sit and stand upright. Standing with both feet firmly on the ground, hands relaxed alongside the body, evokes an experience of being grounded. Standing with the feet apart and hands on the hips reinforces a sense of stability. Standing erect is the first step in learning to stand up for oneself, to stand one's ground.

Being able to sit and stand up straight has another benefit: It enhances the body's capacity to take in a greater amount of oxygen with each breath. An uptick in oxygen helps young people think more clearly and make better decisions (Medina, 2012).

A 2008 study examined incidents of bullying among elementary school children in Boulder, Colorado. The yoga intervention combined philosophy, postures, breathing, and concentration techniques with conflict resolution strategies. Students who participated in the yoga program reported a 60% decrease in their own bullying behaviors, as well as 42% fewer incidents of being bullied by classmates (Marie et al., 2008).

After observing a high school yoga class, I had the opportunity to speak with a student who has changed since beginning school yoga:

> I used to get into lots of fights. I had this urge to hit someone when I got angry. Then I started doing yoga every day in school. I noticed that I felt different in yoga class—quiet inside. Peaceful. When kids said something that I didn't like, usually I would go crazy. Toward the end of the first term, I surprised myself. I started to walk away. I'd smile and think, "Peace begins with me. Peace begins with me." I'm a much happier person now. (personal communication, January 27, 2015)

Donna Davis also sees changes among her yoga students at the large Orlando, Florida, high school where she teaches PE. "A lot of the girls tell me that they are different in their relationships with friends or boyfriends—less likely to say something hurtful or mean. It changes how they interact with others. They reflect more before they speak" (personal communication, April 10, 2015).

Yoga opens young people to a world of possibilities. By practicing mindful movement, focus, and self-calming, students may discover a source of clarity and charity that they did not know they had. In Amy Saltzman's book, *A Still Quiet Place*, she cites the ABCs of classroom mindfulness: A is for attention; B is for breath; and C is for choice. "When we stop and pay attention to our breath, then sometimes we can make . . . a choice that is kind to us and kind to others" (2014, p. 140).

CHAPTER 8

Yoga for Students With Autism Spectrum Disorder and Special Needs

YOGA REDUCES STRESS and promotes imitation, playfulness, and social interaction among a wide range of children. These skills are especially important for many of those with exceptional needs. Providing this instruction in an atmosphere of acceptance, free from judgment or competition, is what makes yoga different from many other forms of exercise. Everyone is included, regardless of physical prowess. Teachers can genuinely praise effort without criticism of form. Any variation of a posture that is safe and comfortable is accepted.

Varied classroom breaks include strength, flexibility, and balance postures. Many yoga routines can be done with students sitting at their desks or using their chairs for support, making it inclusive for children with diverse physical challenges. Often, children in wheelchairs can take part alongside their classmates. Yoga breaks can be short or long, quiet or noisy, silly or contemplative. Because it's literally performed eye to eye—seated, standing, or on the ground— yoga offers students a level playing field among classmates and with their teachers.

Setting a mood with soft lighting and music is often useful to signal the transition to yoga breaks. The calming tone, soft volume, and gentle rhythm of the teacher's voice and a consistent pattern of instruction create a nonmenacing environment for students who are often anxious (see Creating a Ritual in Chapter 16).

According to Children and Adults With Attention Deficit/Hyperactivity Disorder (CHADD), 5–11% of school-age children have symptoms of ADHD. These include challenges in paying attention, following directions, sitting still, and containing impulsivity. "Increasingly, researchers are studying ADHD in the context of executive functions—the brain functions that activate, organize, integrate, and manage other functions. Impairment of these executive functions is considered highly interrelated to symptoms associated with ADHD" (CHADD, 2015).

Shifting attention requires focus. Yoga is an intervention that teaches children how to focus. Students learn to inhabit their bodies in very specific ways when doing a yoga pose. They are instructed where to place each foot and each hand, in what direction to turn the head and where to look with the eyes, when to inhale, and when to exhale. By engaging the mind and body fully in a posture, a student may experience a sense of presence, of being in the moment. This liberation from distraction invites a rare experience of calm for many.

Psychologist Clinton Lewis incorporates yoga into his Oklahoma City practice when working with adolescents with ADHD. He describes the "increased relaxation and physical and emotional awareness through yoga practice, especially for kids who have difficulty managing their behavior in the classroom and with peers. The self-calming they experience increases their awareness of and ability to talk about their feelings. They make different decisions, resisting impulses to act out in class" (personal communication, June 1, 2012).

Yoga instruction affords many opportunities to enhance communication skills and to communicate in varying ways. Poses can be taught using simple one-word instructions, short phrases, or detailed information including anatomy and physiology. Yoga lends itself well to a visual curriculum. Visual cues provide a focal point for students with attention deficits or sensory processing challenges—demonstrating where to stand and where to focus their eyes. They also make postures more accessible to many individuals on the autism spectrum as well as for students with limited access to language.

Cathy Calandriello, ChildLight Yoga teacher and Creative Relaxation practitioner, is an Exceptional Student Education (ESE) teacher at Dover Middle School.

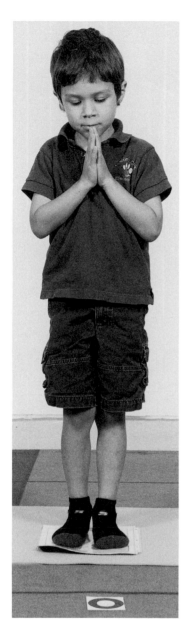

8-1 Focal Point

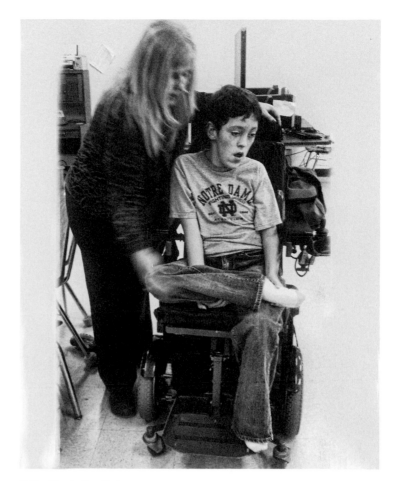

8-2 Rock the Baby

She has offered yoga to ESE classes in this New Hampshire public school since early 2014. I observed her teaching a class for children with diverse challenges, including ASD, ADHD, emotional handicaps, and physical disabilities. Assisted by a classroom paraprofessional, one student joined his classmates in the circle from his wheelchair. Students' faces lit up as they did their favorite postures. In rock the baby pose, children sang and hugged their shins as if lulling a baby to sleep.

Calandriello and Stacey McDonough, a school social worker, use the S.T.O.P. and Relax (Goldberg et al., 2006) visual cues displayed on a flip easel during

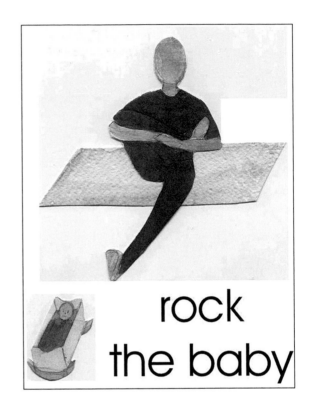

8-3   Visual Cue Card S.T.O.P. and Relax

instruction. Following a visual routine, McDonough explained, mitigates anxiety about what comes next and facilitates imitation. "They can see the picture; they can read the posture name; they can follow along. As the routine becomes more familiar, they feel more comfortable and begin to relax" (personal communication, November 24, 2014).

Both educators have seen changes among the yoga participants. Calandriello notes improved focus, an increase in self-calming behaviors throughout the school day, and a greater willingness to engage in physical exercise. "Now they even come up with their own ideas for poses and activities. And the relationships I've developed with these kids have been helpful for problem solving in other classroom situations and school environments" (personal communication, January 8, 2016).

Many young people need help in learning how to rein themselves in and make thoughtful choices. But children with neurological challenges may have additional difficulties in accessing self-regulation techniques. Individuals with autism tend to have high levels of stress hormones, suggesting that their self-calming mechanism (vagal system) may be dysregulated, according to Dr. Stephen Porges. Self-stimulating activities such as rocking and spinning "may reflect a naturally occurring behavioral strategy to stimulate and regulate a vagal system that is not efficiently functioning" (Porges, 2005, p. 73; see Chapter 10).

A number of yoga positions such as partner rocking and gentle circular motions of the spine promote a calming effect similar to those described by Porges. Guiding students to use these postures has helped avert numerous

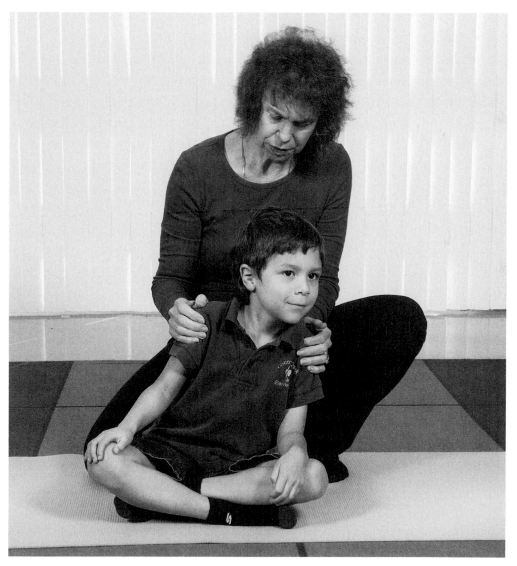

8-4   Seated Circles

meltdowns (Goldberg, 2013). According to Porges, "Since there is now documentation that children with autism . . . do not efficiently regulate . . . the [nervous system] . . . yoga could be an efficient portal to improve this system" (personal communication, July 20, 2012).

In 2001, a group of educators and I conducted a study of six upper elementary school children on the autism spectrum who displayed dysfunction and anxiety under stress (Goldberg, 2004a). Creative Relaxation classes of yoga postures, breathing, guided relaxation, role-playing, and discussion met three times a week for 30-minute periods. Instruction was carried out using the S.T.O.P. and Relax visual curriculum and props (Goldberg et al., 2006).

In addition to practice on yoga mats, a portion of the classes were conducted seated in chairs in a simulated classroom environment. Through modeling and prompting, students learned techniques for generalizing the relaxation techniques they had practiced, responding to verbal cues such as "relax" and

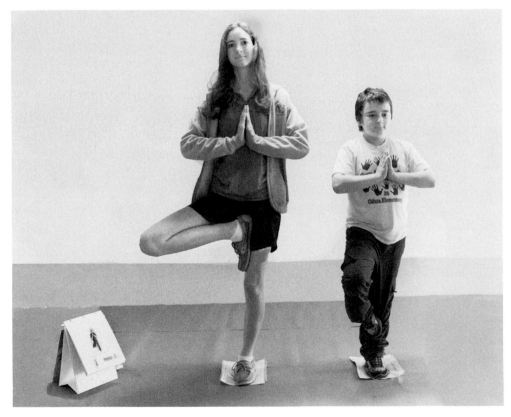

8-5 Easel and Props, S.T.O.P. and Relax

"breathe." "Classroom teachers reported increased alertness . . . and more self-monitoring [and] . . . were able to use the relaxation cues to help children deescalate in volatile situations" (Goldberg, 2004b, p. 77).

Yoga postures can be used for behavior management and lowering frustration levels. Redirecting children before they lose control is key to maintaining order in the classroom and to avoid reinforcing disruptive behaviors. Autism educator Janet Janzen suggests taking a break to help students regain and maintain control:

> Most people automatically know when their stress is so high that they must get out of a situation quickly, and they automatically know how to reduce their stress. . . . But those with autism must be taught positive ways to escape overwhelming stress before they lose control. Even very young children can learn to take a break independently. Taking a break to relieve stress is a positive skill that is taught and reinforced in order to prevent a behavioral problem. This break is very different from a time-out that occurs after losing control. (1996, pp. 358–359)

In yoga breaks, children practice varied forms of stress reduction. Simple tools for readjusting their respiratory and heart rates are explored throughout this text. Postures such as Volcano Squat (Unit 8) and Self-Hug (Unit 6) provide deep touch pressure that is generally soothing to individuals with sensory challenges. Partner rocking is calming and gives children a chance to experience connection through touch.

Not all individuals find comfort in touch, however. Temple Grandin, like many individuals on the autism spectrum, is highly sensitive to touch. Her discomfort with physical contact added to her challenges in relating to others. The family cat ran whenever she would try to hold it because she inadvertently hurt the animal. Grandin devised an apparatus that allowed her to

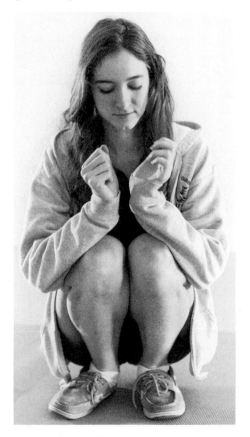

8-6   Volcano Squat

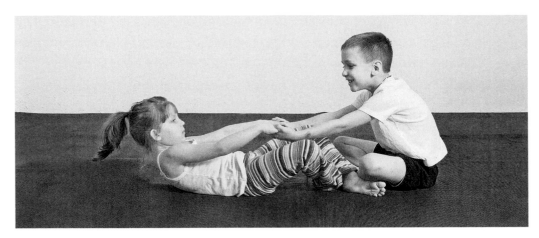

8-7   Partner Seesaw

adjust touch pressure to her own specifications, so it became tolerable to her. As a result, her receptivity to touch from others also increased. She was finally successful in learning to comfort her cat. She explains, "To have feelings of gentleness, one must experience gentle bodily comfort. . . . Gentle touch teaches kindness" (Grandin, 2006, pp. 84–85).

By approaching children at their eye level, as we do in yoga, it's possible to prevent a great deal of defensiveness and anxiety. Respecting boundaries is essential to building trust with those who are highly sensitive to touch. It's important to ask permission before getting close or touching a child, and to learn to interpret the response—especially when dealing with children with speech or language deficits. If there is any doubt that touch is welcome, avoid it.

I have observed many students growing tolerant to touch in yoga classes. Working in a center for students with emotional behavioral disorders, I was surprised when high school students peeled off heavy outer vests and jackets to receive a gentle back massage in Baby pose. Immediately after the posture, they put back all their protective layers—their armor—even in the warm south Florida climate (Goldberg, 2004a).

Many young people with ASD have gradually accepted my invitation to partner in a pose, knowing that it is their choice. In addition, there are alternatives to partner poses that invite connection without physical touch. By working side by side, for example, students can experience partnering without the stress of actual physical contact. They may rest against a wall or chair instead of a person

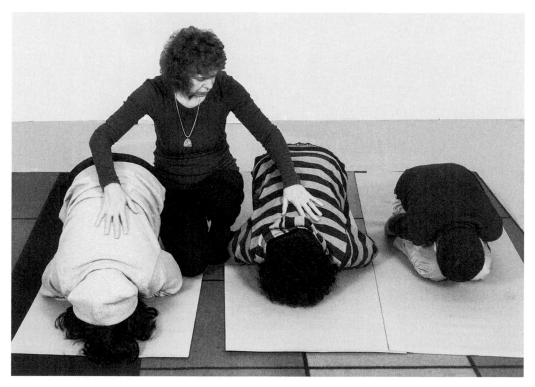

8-8 Massage in Baby Pose

to experience support in a posture. These are tools to help them feel more in control of their own bodies and personal space. As students become accustomed to yoga postures, they may respond to them as transitional prompts between activities. Some students find a favorite pose that is especially soothing or engaging (see Appendix 3). As teachers observe the efficacy of a particular posture or breathing exercise, they may signal the child to use it at intervals throughout the day to assist with self-regulation. Teachers may share the child's personal pose with parents and other professionals, creating a common tool among the student's support team.

You'll find practices and adaptations that are geared toward young people with special needs interspersed throughout this book. The approach is purposefully inclusive, so that students can participate in general education as well as ESE classes at school. Many of the lessons can also be practiced at home with parents and siblings or in therapeutic settings.

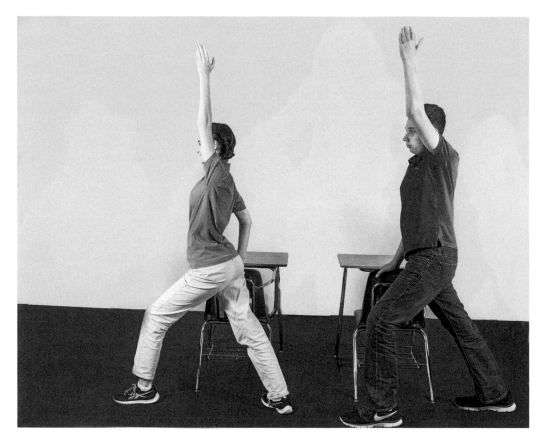

8-9   Desk Support in Warrior

Yoga is exquisitely suited to youths with varying exceptionalities. It lends itself to multiple modalities, combining visual, auditory, kinesthetic, and tactile learning. It promotes playful interaction and eases anxiety. Variations are welcome in every posture. Far more important than how a student performs a pose is how he or she feels in a pose. Finding comfort in yoga breaks is what makes the experience healing for all children.

For many more specific techniques, postures, and routines, please refer to *Yoga Therapy for Children with Autism and Special Needs* (Goldberg, 2013).

CHAPTER 9

Partnering With the School Community: Administration, Teachers, Parents

W HEN LEADING TEACHER training in Creative Relaxation yoga, one question frequently arises: How do I get a yoga program started in my school? In my experience as an educational consultant, there have been three primary avenues for bringing yoga into classrooms: administrators, teachers, and parents.

Sometimes it's advantageous to start at the top. After I volunteered to demonstrate yoga's benefits to the staff of a center for children with emotional, behavioral, and neurological disorders in 1981, the visionary principal, John Smith, hired me to provide direct instruction to students K–12. Collecting data— your own or that of other professionals—to validate the effectiveness of yoga can also be highly effective. A simple study measuring students' pulse rates before and after yoga practice over a period of 8 weeks (Goldberg, 2004b) was sufficient to expand a fledgling yoga project county-wide in 2001. By graphing the results of the pulse rate study, parent questionnaires, and teacher observation, my colleagues and I earned the endorsement of a district curriculum specialist to continue funding our program.

Classroom teachers are crucial in this process. Many whom I've worked with have received funding for training and materials directly through their administration. Others have applied for modest grants from the school district, local banks, and national organizations to bring in trainers and outfit their classrooms with materials. A key component of the most successful grant recipients' projects has been training the classroom teacher to carry on the yoga program after the training period has been completed.

A third avenue for bringing yoga into schools has been parents. Donna Davis's yoga program at Edgewater High was initiated by a parent volunteer. Many parent groups—PTA, PTO—have funded small yoga projects and material acquisitions in my local districts. The ESE Advisory Board in the Broward Schools has supported ongoing family yoga programs and parent stress reduction presentations.

Getting yoga in the door is only the first step. Engaging the administration, teachers, and parents in yoga instruction is often what makes the difference between another great idea and a lasting, successful school program.

Of course, none of this matters without student buy-in. In a report on implementing mindfulness and yoga in school settings, Mendelson and colleagues discussed the importance of a partnership among administrators, teachers, and students:

> School administrative support—namely, commitment from the principal, vice principal and other leaders in the school—was identified . . . as critical for successful programme implementation. Active administrative involvement with the intervention communicated to teachers and students that the school valued and was committed to the programme and that it should be taken seriously. . . . Small gestures on the part of administrative personnel often had large impacts on student motivation. (2013, p. 279)

Occasional visits to classes by principals, for example, improved student behavior and increased motivation.

Teachers are key for program success: "Whereas the administration sets the tone and expectation of what a school will do to support the programme, teachers [are] responsible for making sure it happens" (Mendelson et al., 2013, p. 280).

The researchers found a correlation between teachers' support for the program and student attendance, punctuality, and commitment.

Engaging the Administration

Alan Johnson is the superintendent of Woodland Hills School District outside Pittsburgh, Pennsylvania, a diverse urban community. Speaking at the Kripalu Yoga in Schools Symposium on April 24, 2014, he stated, "To get yoga into school, you have to be a solution to a problem. That's what administrators will pursue."

In his district, an area of great need was the alternative education center for students with emotional and behavioral challenges. With behavior problems rampant, Johnson was receptive to allocating funds and energy to improve the program. A yoga educator from the Yoga in Schools program was brought in to train the teachers, behavioral specialists, and staff to implement yoga in their school.

Johnson reported, "It's been phenomenal. Fights, weapons on campus, severe behavioral disruptions went from being daily or weekly events to this: from Thanksgiving through late April [2014], there has not been a single event." Based on data collected to validate the conditions for success of the program in his district, he stressed the importance of school-wide engagement, especially among the teachers. This was facilitated by the top-down approach to yoga education: "Data showed that in buildings where there was good buy-in by the school community, there was a reduction in disruption and behaviors."

Lisa Flynn, founder of Yoga 4 Classrooms, has been supporting schools in integrating yoga and mindfulness into the school day for over 10 years:

Ownership and sustainability comes only when the school is internally invested, when they take the reins and make the program their own. Unfortunately, unless the administration is mandating implementation, just as they would any other new curricular initiative, it will not be sustainable. In our experience, strong leadership, teaming, proper training, and long-term support are the keys to school-wide implementation and success. (personal communication, September 19, 2015)

Engaging Teachers

Like Lisa Flynn, I have found the best results in school programs when the initiative comes from the administration. However, as Superintendent Alan Johnson said, "It's the teachers that make it happen."

When the school yoga program is mandated by the administration, it's especially important to consider the needs and reservations of the classroom teachers who will be carrying it out. My colleagues at S.T.O.P. and Relax and I have had opportunities to address this challenge.

During the 2014–2015 school year, the Mailman Segal Center at Nova Southeastern University received a grant from Autism Speaks to implement our school yoga program in the curriculum at the Baudhuin Preschool. Located in south Florida, Baudhuin is an internationally recognized model program for children with ASD.

Inspired by school director Nancy Lieberman, the objectives were to outfit each classroom with teaching materials, train the faculty to implement the curriculum, and provide resources for school families.

Although most were enthusiastic, some teachers were understandably put off by the prospect of adding another demand on their time. To lessen the burden, we developed a series of short training modules that fit during after-school prep time and on early release days. The first program was inclusive of all staff, which is especially important when the program is generated by outside providers. By clarifying the objectives, terminology, and research-based methodology for the yoga program, we increased the likelihood of buy-in from teachers and support staff. In addition, we better equipped them to answer questions from families.

Instructional modules combined discussion and movement, so the teachers experienced the playful and relaxing benefits of yoga. At the teachers' request, we eliminated a big time consumer in preschool by having children practice with shoes on. Teachers were encouraged to add just one S.T.O.P. and Relax activity into their schedules to start. Posture adaptations were provided for students with limited motor skills. To address the varied attention skills of the students, we offered visual lessons ranging from as brief as 1 minute to as long as a 20-minute class period.

After the training modules were completed, I had the opportunity to visit classrooms to offer on-site coaching. I was amazed at the innovative approaches I observed. Some teachers had added a single breathing technique and one posture as part of their daily circle time. Others practiced poses with children sitting in their chairs. One classroom had a yoga area with the visuals of the day's yoga sequence posted on the wall. Several teachers had divided the students into yoga groups, rotating them with other activities within the classroom. Some lessons were brief; others lasted 10 or 20 minutes and contained all the elements of a full class.

It was extraordinary to see the level of engagement of these preschoolers. Their teachers shared countless examples of children responding to the instruction in positive ways.

Seeing the benefits of the program had been highly motivating for the teachers—so much so that every classroom teacher implemented some aspect of yoga into her curriculum. School director Nancy Lieberman reported, "The S.T.O.P. and Relax program has exceeded my expectations. Not only in terms of the teachers, some of whom I was not sure would take to it. But the students demonstrate every day that this program has a place in our curriculum" (personal communication, May 16, 2015).

Engaging Parents

Middle school is a place where emotions frequently run high. A veteran middle school principal who has implemented a yoga program in her school shared the positive response from parents. "They have observed the calming effect and the sense of community that yoga brings to this age group. The kids tell me how much they love having yoga at the end of their school day, so they leave school feeling more peaceful. Parents notice this, too. We all see the way kids support each other in yoga. One sixth grader really blossomed in the class. Another child who doesn't fit in much with the other kids in school has found a fit in yoga. It's a safe place for these and many others. Parents appreciate how this affects their children" (personal communication, December 15, 2014).

When I first began teaching yoga in schools, nearly 35 years ago, most parents and educators didn't know much about yoga or its intent. This influenced numerous aspects of Creative Relaxation, my school yoga curriculum. It includes child-friendly names for all of the postures. There are no Sanskrit words or chants.

Instead of "Namaste," class begins with, "Hello, friends." There is plenty of singing in posture, but no Sanskrit prayers. Instead of chanting om, we sing vowel sounds like oh and ah to extend the exhalation. Rather than salutations to the sun, we reach high to the sun and low to the ground.

Each time I start at a new school, we offer an open house for parents to ask questions and experience a sample lesson. It's important for families to see for themselves that the school program is completely secular and to have a forum to voice concerns.

While implementing the yoga program at the Baudhuin Preschool, we provided a morning session (with continental breakfast) for parents that included an informative presentation, video taken of the children doing poses in their classes, and a gentle yoga experience. This freed the teachers from having to respond to many of the questions about the program, while engaging the community in the project. Several parents shared stories of seeing their children practicing Huh Breaths (see Unit 1) on their own and wondering what they had been doing. Parents welcomed the suggestions they received for home practice. In addition to helping their families, this reinforced the work of the classroom teachers.

Educating parents and teachers about what yoga is and what it is not may mitigate a great deal of potential misunderstanding and tension. The families involved in the Encinitas, California, court case against their school yoga program had never been to their child's class to observe the yoga practice, according to Superintendent Timothy Baird at Kripalu Yoga in Schools Symposium, 2014.

One Pennsylvania PE teacher recommends making the yoga curriculum available to all parents. When a family objected to the inclusion of yoga in PE, the teacher invited them in to watch as many classes as they wanted. To their credit, they came to school to see for themselves. After showing them his curriculum, including a visual representation of all the

9-1   Huh Breath

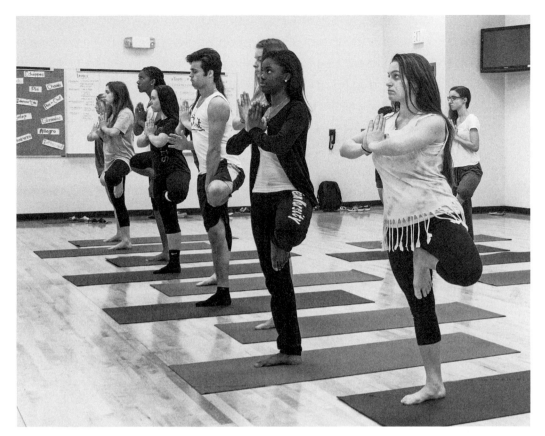

9-2 Tree Hands

postures, he asked them to select any positions that they wanted eliminated from their child's class program. In this case, once they saw exactly what school yoga was, their concerns were quelled.

In response to another family's objections, one teacher explained that yoga was an essential part of the football team's workout. The teacher didn't feel the team would be as well-balanced, focused, and protected from injury by other workout routines. Discovering that ending yoga might interfere with the school football program, the family rescinded their request.

Teachers have told me that occasionally families object to the hand position with the palms together, thumbs at the sternum. I call this Tree Hands, but it is sometimes called prayer position. I have found it helpful to explain the rationale for this hand position: Placing the hands at the center of the chest helps students focus on their breathing, feeling the subtle movement in their palms with inhalation and exhalation. It also brings their awareness to the muscles in the front of the chest and mid-back, involved in respiration and necessary for standing or sitting upright. Nonetheless, it's easy to make adaptations with hand positions. For example, students may rest the hands on the belly or alongside the thighs, or they may interlace the fingers behind the back. When teachers acknowledge and respond to parents' concerns, most families support school yoga.

With its current popularity, yoga is embraced by many parents and school personnel today. There are programs that include Sanskrit terminology, much like any other language taught in a classroom. Saying namaste and chanting om are an integral part of some school curricula. In my experience, however, I have found it advisable to omit anything that might be construed as nonsecular when initiating a school yoga program.

The onus is on the yoga educator to create a program that is acceptable to all families, to welcome parents' comments, and to honor their concerns. As yoga psychologist Laura Douglass cautions, neither advocates nor opponents to school yoga are served by simply dismissing opposing viewpoints. Rather, she encourages a thoughtful, intellectual dialogue that is consistent with the cultural diversity within our democratic educational system (Douglass, 2010).

PART III

NEUROSCIENCE MEETS YOGA

At the intersection between biology and psychology, a new field . . . [is] emerging called social neuroscience. It's the study of how our nervous system affects the way we interact with one another and how we express emotions like empathy and compassion. At the center of several studies in this field are yoga and meditation, ancient practices that are gaining new life. (Chopra et al., 2015)

CHAPTER 10

Stress, Learning, and the Adolescent Brain

Y OU'VE PROBABLY AWAKENED to the startling sound of a telephone call in the middle of the night. It's hard not to imagine that something awful has happened. In that moment, your heart starts pounding, your breathing becomes shallow; your hands are clammy when you grab for the phone. Even if the call is to let you know that all is well—your son decided to stay at a friend's for the night; your daughter's baby was born a week early—it may take hours to shake off the effects of that intrusion on your nervous system.

Let's explore why this happens.

The Limbic System

As neuroendocrinologist Bruce McEwen states, "Stress begins in the brain" (2002, p. 34). Although our bodies and the types of stressors have changed significantly since prehistoric times, the manner in which we respond to danger—whether real or imagined—hasn't changed much at all (Selye, 1974). In fact, it's our perception of stress—what we infer through our senses and past experience—that activates the nervous system. In other words, worrying about a possible calamity may take the same bodily toll as actually experiencing the calamity.

The limbic system, sometimes referred to as the emotional center of the brain, has two structures prominently involved in the stress process: the amygdala and the hippocampus. These also are essential for higher functions of the brain, including learning and memory (McEwen, 2002). The amygdala, described by Joseph LeDoux (1996) as the "low road," reacts immediately to possible danger by tripping the internal panic button, initiating the stress response (McEwen, 2002). It bypasses the reasoning center located at the front of the brain above the eyes, the prefrontal cortex, or the "high road" (LeDoux, 1996). The amygdala also transmits instructions to the prefrontal cortex to assess the current threat, but it doesn't wait for the brain's executive capacities to mull things over before activating the fight-or-flight response (van der Kolk, 2014). This rapid response is essential for survival.

The other structure involved in this process is the hippocampus. In addition to forming new memories, it organizes and stores information, creating a sort of filing system for cross-referencing and disposing of unneeded data (McEwen, 2002). When the amygdala perceives a threat, the hippocampus compares it to past experiences; this helps the amygdala determine whether to sound the stress alarm (van der Kolk, 2014).

The Autonomic Nervous System

The nervous system is the body's communication network, gathering information from the environment for processing through the brain. The autonomic nervous system (ANS), a division of the peripheral nervous system, is tasked with maintaining the functioning of the heart, blood vessels, respiration, endocrine and immune systems, digestion, and elimination. Two complementary components work together in the ANS to maintain internal balance, also known as homeostasis. The sympathetic nervous system (SNS) accelerates internal activity in response to stress—fight or flight; the parasympathetic nervous system (PNS), sometimes called "rest and digest," restores the internal equilibrium.

When stress triggers the internal alarm, the nervous system makes a quick shift to sympathetic dominance. This accelerates the heart rate and respiration, rushes blood to the limbs, and floods the system with adrenaline, increasing resilience in addressing the threat to body or mind. Known as allostasis, it is this system that keeps the body stable and functioning while supporting the demands made upon it (McEwen, 2002). After the crisis, the brain receives the signal to cancel the stress response, and the body returns to normal functioning.

Imagine a little boy and a little girl of approximately the same size on a see-saw. They ride gently up and down, with ease. That's comparable to homeostasis—a balancing act between the sympathetic and parasympathetic divisions of the ANS.

One day the girl brings her backpack loaded with her lunchbox, five heavy school books, and three bottles of water. After her friend mounts the seesaw, she takes her seat wearing the heavy pack. At once, the movement becomes erratic. Weighed down at her end, the little girl tries to push and force her way up. If she gets off suddenly, the boy will plummet. If she doesn't, no matter how hard the boy thrashes and kicks, he can't get down.

Stranded at the top of the seesaw, the boy begins to panic. A sick feeling starts in his stomach and creeps up the back of his neck. His amygdala sounds the alarm. His breathing becomes shallow and rapid and his heart is pounding. The amygdala has alerted his adrenal glands to release epinephrine (adrenaline), rushing blood to his limbs, increasing his strength. He kicks and strains, but he cannot overcome the imbalanced conditions.

During brief bouts of stress, there is also an increase of the neurotransmitter dopamine, which "sharpens and focuses the mind" (Ratey, 2008, p. 64). In a moment of clarity, the little boy assesses the situation. "Throw off your back-pack!" he calls to the confused little girl at the bottom, watching helplessly as her friend struggles to get down. She shrugs the pack off, and immediately the see-saw levels. Within seconds, both children dismount and catch their breath. After a rest, they are back on the seesaw—no backpacks—laughing and joking. All is well.

Prolonged Stress: HPA Axis and Cortisol

During extended periods of stress, the body calls in additional reserves. Information passes from the amygdala to the hypothalamus to the pituitary gland, activating the hypothalamic-pituitary-adrenal (HPA) axis (McEwen, 2002).

This incites the release of the second wave of stress hormones, cortisol, a glucocorticoid. To increase energy reserves, the body begins converting muscle to fat (stored around the waist during long bouts with stress) and extracting minerals from bones (McEwen, 2002). The HPA axis keeps the heart, brain, and muscle tissue in a state of high alert while slowing the digestive and reproductive systems. In addition, prolonged stress compromises the immune system.

When the brain gets the all-clear sign, cortisol serves an additional function: It signals the hypothalamus to shut down the stress circuit. The body now begins the process of repairing and rebalancing.

Stress changes the brain in a number of ways. Chronic stress can impair the body's ability to switch off stress responses, even during periods of calm. It also can increase the reactivity of the amygdala (Bremner et al., 2008), setting off the panic button more frequently. Prolonged stress can affect cognition, behavior, and mental health (Lupien et al., 2009) and may lead to depression (Streeter et al., 2012). Neuroendocrinologist Robert Sapolsky (2003) notes the negative impact of stress on sleep and mood cycles due to a decrease in serotonin levels.

As previously mentioned, the amygdala and hippocampus play a crucial role in learning and memory; stress-related changes to the brain interfere with these higher functions (McEwen, 2002).

Stress and Learning

Stress is disruptive to the learning process. Research has shown that periods of peak learning coincide with an increase in the number of new brain cells (neurogenesis) in the hippocampus, increasing its size (Maguire et al., 2000). In contrast, prolonged periods of stress have been shown to reduce the size of the hippocampus (Gage, 2003).

A small amount of stress from a reasonable challenge—what Sapolsky (2003, p. 93) describes as "stimulation"—elevates the feel-good neurotransmitter dopamine. Excessive stress, however, interrupts this flow, curbing the pleasant feelings.

Neurologist and educator Judy Willis (2014) explains that stressed-out students cannot absorb new information: "Additional neuroimaging studies of the amygdala, hippocampus, and the rest of the limbic system, along with measurement of dopamine and other brain chemical transmitters during the learning process, reveal that students' comfort level has a critical impact on information transmission and storage in the brain."

Yoga, when integrated into the school curriculum, has been shown to lower levels of cortisol. Butzer, Day, and colleagues (2015) explored the impact of a 10-week Yoga 4 Classrooms intervention on levels of stress hormones in second and third grade students. The second graders who participated in the program had a significant decrease in baseline cortisol after the intervention. In addition, the second-grade teacher perceived significant improvements in academic and SEL competencies, including interaction among classmates, the ability to attend, concentrate, and stay on task, and academic achievement. These students also exhibited improved stress management, lowered anxiety, increased confidence, and improved mood. Grade two and three students demonstrated increased creativity, better behavior control, and improved anger management (Butzer, Day, et al., 2015).

The Adolescent Brain

Teenagers live life more intensely than younger children and adults. They are prone to quick reflexes and impulsive behaviors. Part of the problem is the state of the limbic system, which becomes "turbo-boosted" in puberty, explains NIMH neuroscientist Jay N. Giedd (2015). Meanwhile, connections to the prefrontal cortex, the part of the brain that makes careful decisions and postpones gratification for long-term gains, are still under construction: "Indeed, we now know that the prefrontal cortex continues to change prominently until well into a person's 20s. And yet puberty seems to be starting earlier, extending the 'mismatch years'" (Giedd, 2015, p. 34).

Giedd (2015, p. 34) describes the exceptional plasticity of the teen brain as a "double-edged sword." While permitting extraordinary gains in their capacity for independent thinking and social interaction, the rapid changes within their brains also make teens more vulnerable to reckless behaviors and serious psychiatric disorders.

Neurologist Frances E. Jensen notes that girls and boys have different growth rates in the brain. The frontal and parietal lobes, both significant in "cognitive maturity," peak in female brains in the early teens but not until the late teens in males (Jensen, 2015, p. 59). The maturation process may continue in male brains through age 30, according to Jensen.

It's not all good news for girls, though. It appears that levels of the stress hormone cortisol, which are higher in teens than in adults, are even higher in mid- to late-adolescent girls than in boys (Jensen, 2015). This may explain the intensified emotions and highs and lows to which adolescent girls seem especially susceptible.

Addressing Anxiety

High cortisol levels and less activity in the prefrontal cortex also complicate a teen's response to stress (Jensen, 2015). Young people are more easily and frequently set off by events that may seem trivial to adult observers: a boy who is devastated after being rejected for a date, even after the girl he sought had refused all advances; a bright student who is convinced that she will fail an exam. Attempts to reassure an anxious teen that there's nothing to worry about or that these feelings will pass fall short. Although their thinking may be faulty, logic provides little comfort.

According to the book *Rewire Your Anxious Brain*, "when you try to use thinking processes and logic to cope with feelings of anxiety, you're relying on cortex-based methods. And by itself, the cortex can't reduce the stress response for two primary reasons. First . . . the cortex doesn't have many direct connections to the amygdala. Second, the initiator of the stress response is the amygdala. . . . Therefore, interventions that target the amygdala are more direct and effective in easing anxiety" (Pittman & Karle, 2015, p. 95).

Simply telling a distraught youth to relax during the throes of fight-or-flight arousal is ineffective. When the nervous system is careening out of control like a car heading off a cliff, the trajectory has to be changed and the brakes applied with great care. Fortunately, interventions such as yoga (Froeliger et al., 2012), breathing exercises (Goldin & Gross 2010), and breathing-focused meditation have been shown to lower activation of the amygdala (Desbordes et al., 2012). "When you reduce amygdala activation, you reduce SNS responding, and with practice, the PNS can be trained to intervene" (Pittman & Karle, 2015, p. 96).

In addition, studies on mindfulness meditation reported increased density in the hippocampus, involved in learning and remembering, and decreased density in the amygdala, the fear and alarm center (Hölzel et al., 2011). "Many of these approaches almost immediately reduce activation in the amygdala. . . . Individuals respond in different ways to various relaxation strategies, but virtually everyone will benefit from relaxation training . . . such as meditation and yoga" (Pittman & Karle, 2015, pp. 96–97).

Clearly, it's very difficult for many young people to talk themselves into feeling safe and calm. Breathing and meditation have been shown to be effective tools for self-calming. These techniques can be taught to youth of all ages, as you'll see throughout this text.

I work with many students, however, who do not have mastery over their breathing or who lack the capacity to sit for meditation. For these individuals, changing their body position is a more effective tool.

I often find that it's easier to let the body breathe the child, so to speak, than to ask the child to change her breathing. Fortunately, many yoga postures are well suited to triggering a calming response. Tucking the chin into the throat notch in a forward bend, for example, increases pressure to the baroreceptors, lowering heart rate and blood pressure (Robin, 2009). Baroreceptors are pressure-sensitive neurons that monitor blood pressure in the throat and other areas of the body (Tortora & Grabowski, 1996). These types of neck flexion generally slow the rate of respiration. Slow twisting, rocking, and circling motions have a similar effect on breathing. Light pressure on the eyebrows or forehead is also calming (Cole, 2008).

Many young people find it easier to move into feelings of quiet and safety than to be talked into those experiences. Stephen Porges agrees "that movement [is] a more effective intervention than talking for calming children. Movement recruits bottom-up signals to the brain stem to trigger brain to body regulatory processes;.. this is more efficient than cortical to brain stem to visceral pathways" (personal communication, June 5, 2015).

According to professor of psychiatry Dan Siegel, "The flow of energy and information from the body up into the cortex changes our bodily states, our emotional states, and our thoughts. . . . The next time your children need help calming down or regaining control, look for ways to get them moving" (2011, p. 59).

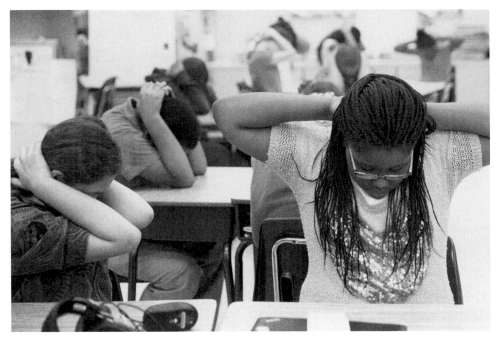

10-1   Chin Tuck

Many of these tools for combating the impact of stress can be implemented in the classroom via short yoga breaks. Moreover, movement is often more accessible to kids than figurative concepts such as "relax your body" or "slow down your breathing." For this reason, each unit of the BREATHE FIRST curriculum includes seated and standing postures, in addition to breathing and focusing lessons. With consistent practice, children can become accomplished at reducing their levels of stress.

Respiration and the Autonomic Nervous System

Your ANS makes a slight shift with every breath: Inhalation is energizing, activating the SNS; exhalation is calming, activating the PNS (Robin, 2009). Believe it or not, this irregularity in the heart rate is a good thing. Called heart rate variability or respiratory sinus arrhythmia (Porges, 2005), greater variations of these rhythms are a sign of good health (Robin, 2009). "In healthy individuals, inhalations and exhalations produce steady, rhythmical fluctuations in heart rate," reflecting a more responsive ANS and a greater capacity to control our responses to minor sources of stress (van der Kolk, 2014, p. 267).

Heart rate and respiration are functions of the ANS, in that they do not require conscious participation. But we also have the ability to change our breathing voluntarily. Breath awareness and control are essential components of yoga. According to research by van der Kolk and colleagues (2014), yoga can improve heart rate variability. In his work with individuals with PTSD, van der Kolk found that "yoga significantly improved arousal problems in PTSD and dramatically improved our subjects' relationships with their bodies" (2014, p. 270).

The reactions of the SNS are linked, so that if one of them is activated, they all become activated, creating a cascade of stress responses, explains yoga scholar Mel Robin (2009). Fortunately, the PNS does not react in the same way. If even one bodily function can be shifted from sympathetic to parasympathetic, this can switch off most or all of the stress responses (Robin, 2009). Slowing down the rate of respiration is an example of this process.

Physicians from University Hospital, Augusta, Georgia, have explored the use of self-regulated breathing and breathing-focused meditation techniques as a primary treatment for anxiety and stress-related disorders. Jerath, Crawford, Barnes, and Harden (2015) suggest addressing the whole body, rather than treating these disorders with medications that alter chemicals in the brain alone. Noting the capacity of respiration to influence emotions and of emotions to alter respiration, they cite breathing and meditation techniques as easy and cost-effective alternatives to pharmacological treatments.

Respiration, the portal between voluntary and involuntary functions, is a highly accessible system. As Porges (2011) explains, slow exhalation effects a change in the heart rate and promotes calm. Increasing the duration of the exhalation enhances healing and well-being. Doubling the exhalation relative to the duration of the inhalation shifts the nervous system into parasympathetic dominance, except during periods of extreme activity or agitation (Coulter, 2001). This underscores the importance of teaching these techniques as yoga breaks during periods of calm throughout the school day.

Yoga and GABA

Gamma-aminobutyric acid (GABA) is a tranquilizing neurotransmitter produced by the brain that reduces anxiety and enhances immunity under stress (Abdou et al., 2006, p. 201). Research at Boston University School of Medicine has demonstrated that yoga increases levels of GABA (Streeter et al., 2007) more effectively than walking (Streeter et al., 2010). The yoga intervention resulted in "acute increases in thalamic GABA levels . . . greater improvement in mood and greater decreases in anxiety" (Streeter et al., 2010, p. 1145).

Streeter's research team "hypothesized that yoga-based practices correct underactivity of the PNS and GABA system in part through stimulation of the vagal nerves, and reduce allostatic load resulting in symptom relief" (2012, p. 571). The higher GABA levels and changes to the HPA axis (which is activated during prolonged periods of stress) brought about through yoga practice make it an effective intervention for reducing stress, pain, and symptoms of PTSD (Streeter et al., 2012).

Elevated GABA levels are also concurrent with feelings of comfort and relaxation, which promote learning readiness and overall calm (Walsh, 2012).

Vagal Influence

It's hard to imagine driving your car without a good set of brakes. Fortunately, your body also comes equipped with a control mechanism that neuroscientist Stephen Porges (2011) calls the "polyvagal brake."

The vagus is the longest of the cranial nerves, spanning from the brain stem at the base of the skull through the belly. Containing afferent (sensory) and efferent (motor) fibers, it influences functions including speech, respiration, heart rate, and digestion (Tortora & Grabowski, 1996). In addition, it helps reset the ANS from stress mode to rest and digest. The sensory nerves of the vagus, explains Porges, inhibit "the HPA axis and reduce cortisol secretion, . . . slow heart rate, lower blood pressure, and reduce arousal to promote calm" (2005, p. 75).

This response is much like the brakes in your car when you are driving downhill. To slow down the vehicle, you keep your foot on the brake. To accelerate, you ease up on the brake. Alternating between the two, you maintain a steady, controlled speed.

"The effective polyvagal brake lets up just enough to activate the sympathetic nervous system when needed, while preventing the body from full fight-or-flight mode at every stressful juncture. A person without a vagal brake lives in an unending state of emergency" (McEwen, 2002, p. 74). A dysregulated vagus, one that does not effectively turn off the fight-or-flight response as needed, renders an individual compromised in retaining or regaining calm. "The vagal afferents exert a powerful regulatory influence on several systems—including . . . pain thresholds, the HPA axis, and the immune system" (Porges, 2005, pp. 75–76). Fortunately, there are ways to activate a sluggish vagal brake.

Simple movements can bring about significant changes, according to Porges: "Shifting posture is a simple way to 'exercise' the . . . vagal circuit via blood pressure afferent (baroreceptors). In fact, I have speculated that many of the benefits of exercise are solely due to posture shifts and challenges to the baroreceptors. This system will respond with a couple of minutes of 'exercise,' which could be as simple as repeatedly sitting and standing" (personal communication, June 5, 2015).

Conclusion

Stress is not a bad thing—moderate challenge and stimulation activate the growth of new cells and connections within the brain. Prolonged periods of stress, however, can deplete the body's reserves and interfere with the learning process. Adolescence, a period of extraordinary brain growth (plasticity), is characterized by intensified emotional responses. The connections from the emotional centers of the brain (limbic system) to the prefrontal cortex, where thoughtful choices are formed, are under construction well beyond the teen years (Giedd, 2015). This helps explain why logical explanations may not be effective at mitigating anxiety in young people. Interventions directed to the limbic system, such as yoga exercises and breathing, have been shown to reduce amygdala activation (Pittman & Karle, 2015), lower levels of stress hormones (Butzer, Day, et al., 2015), and elevate the body's natural tranquilizing agent (Streeter et al., 2010).

As Porges explains, movement triggers receptors in the body to lower blood pressure and slow the heart rate. Changing body positions and using specific types of movement aid the body in activating its internal mechanism to regulate the stress response. The vagal brake can shift the nervous system from fight or flight and help it attain a more balanced rhythm—conducive to learning and responsible social interactions.

CHAPTER 11

Children Need to Move

SCHOOL IS A full-time job for kids. They are required to sit for hours on end, absorb facts and figures that may have little relevance to their daily lives, and take home heavy workloads that consume the meager leisure time left in their day. It's difficult enough for those students who are highly motivated; for many others, the school routine becomes intolerable.

During a conversation with a school counselor, a school nurse, and a high school senior, an interesting question arose: What keeps the average high school kid from succeeding in school? The response was unanimous: boredom. School social worker Rich Foss agrees with this assessment. "Kids in school are bored out of their minds. Most of what they are learning is unimportant to them. Because of the media-rich world that they live in, they have very little patience. They would rather watch than read—it's more stimulating and requires far fewer steps. Most kids would rather do interactive, hands-on activities—anything except sit and take notes all day" (personal communication, September 17, 2015).

In fact, excessive sitting causes weakness in the postural muscles (the ones that hold you erect) and inordinate tension in the neck, shoulders, lower back, and pelvis. In a *Washington Post* blog, pediatric occupational therapist Angela

Hanscom explains the perils of too little movement for children: "Bodies start to succumb to these unnatural positions and sedentary lifestyle through atrophy of the muscles, tightness of ligaments (where there shouldn't be tightness), and underdeveloped sensory systems—setting them up for weak bodies, poor posturing, and inefficient sensory processing of the world around them" (Strauss, 2014).

According to the Centers for Disease Control and Prevention (CDC, 2015b), even moderate exercise increases strength and improves endurance, builds stronger bones and muscles, maintains weight, lowers stress and anxiety levels, elevates self-esteem, and may help regulate blood pressure and cholesterol levels. In addition, regular physical activity may contribute to improved school performance, including better grades, behavior, concentration, and attentiveness to schoolwork (CDC, 2015b). Conversely, childhood and adolescent inactivity can lead to obesity, diabetes, and cardiovascular disease in adulthood (CDC, 2015b).

Even so, the CDC reported that in 2013, fewer than half of students in high school attended physical education classes during an average week (2015b). A Kaiser study found that school-aged kids spend an average of 7½ hours a day in front of some sort of screen—playing video games, scanning the Internet, watching movies—seven days a week: "Moreover, since young people spend so much of that time using two or more media concurrently, they are actually exposed to more than 10½ hours . . . of media content during that period. And this does *not* include time spent using the computer for school work, or time spent texting or talking on a cell phone" (Rideout et al., 2010, p. 11).

Most scientists agree that people are not meant to be immobile. John Medina reminds us in *Brain Rules* that our ancestors walked many miles each day, hunted, fished, and used their bodies to survive. Movement, he believes, is essential for physical and mental well-being: "Cutting off physical exercise—the very activity most likely to promote cognitive performance—to do better on a test score is like trying to gain weight by starving yourself. A smarter approach would be to insert more, not less, exercise into the daily curriculum" (Medina, 2014, p. 33).

Time Well Spent

Despite the growing body of literature that demonstrates improved concentration, behavior, and focus among schoolchildren who practice yoga and other forms of exercise during their school day (Conboy et al., 2013; Frank et al., 2014; Gothe et al., 2013; Mendelson et al., 2010), educators are always concerned about taking time away from schoolwork. After an extensive review of the literature on physical activity and its relationship to academic outcomes for schoolchildren, pediatrician and U.C. San Diego Medical School professor Howard Taras concluded that "physical activities programs help children develop social skills, improve mental health, and reduce risk-taking behaviors. . . . There is evidence to suggest that short-term cognitive benefits of physical activity during the school day adequately compensate for time spent away from other academic areas" (2005, p. 218).

In his book *Brain-Based Learning: The New Paradigm of Teaching*, Eric Jensen (2008) encourages the use of "slow stretching and breathing exercises to increase circulation and oxygen flow to the brain" and movement breaks every 20 minutes. Jensen envisions a classroom where students are free to stand, stretch, or move as they feel the need, in order to "monitor or manage their energy levels" (pp. 38–39).

According to the Pearson Index of cognitive skills and educational attainment, Finland's schools have ranked in the top five in the world for most of the 21st century. Yet Finnish students have shorter school days, less homework, and more time to play, according to *Smithsonian* magazine (Hancock, 2011). Students receive a 15-minute break—personal time—at the end of each instructional period. They can play games, go outside, read, chat, or do nothing. That may seem like a lot of wasted time in a day, but statistics reflect that this is time well spent.

Chicago high school teacher Sophia Faridi describes the importance of taking a break from the intensity of classroom studies, based on her observations in Finnish schools: "Finns believe that students' capacity for engagement and learning is most successful when they have a chance to unwind and refocus. In turn, students work productively during class time, with the understanding that their needs to play, talk, or even read quietly will be met shortly" (Faridi, 2014).

Psychobiologist Jaak Panksepp is an expert on the relationship between play and learning. His research in this field spans three decades. He is a proponent of physical play and movement breaks during the school day to facilitate learning: "Anything to give free quality-fun time for each 40–50 minutes of instruction is bound to have great benefits for children's happiness as well as their capacity to attend to subsequent lessons (if the Finnish experience is any guide)." Panksepp suggested 10 minutes of play followed by a 5-minute calming session to reduce stress (personal communication, March 1, 2015).

Regular "brain rests" during the school day prevent fatigue and frustration, according to Judy Willis, who is both a neurologist and an elementary school teacher. She recommends movement, stretching, or other relaxing activities. There is only so much information that can be consumed at one time, she explains, and some children need rest as often as every 15 minutes to maintain the intensity required during a busy school day. "When a child is not alert and focused, no amount of repetition will drive the information into his memory storage banks" (Willis, 2008, p. 23).

Biologist and educator Carla Hannaford (2005) explored the relationship between learning and movement in her book *Smart Moves*. She shared stories of children with severe learning challenges who made extraordinary academic and social leaps, once liberated from the "sitting still, being quiet, and memorizing" approach to education (Hannaford, 2005, p. 13). She implemented 2-minute breathing Brain Gym breaks to foster self-regulation, reinforcing her "conviction that movement, play, and interpersonal connection was somehow essential to learning" (p. 20).

"Our brain structure is intimately connected to and grown by the movement mechanisms within our body," explains Hannaford (2005, p. 16). Harvard professor John Ratey shares this position: "Exercise influences learning directly, at the cellular level, improving the brain's potential to log in and process new information" (Ratey, 2008, p. 35).

In fact, exercise has been shown to improve executive function—the ability to plan, schedule, switch tasks, and stay focused while in a highly stimulating environment, according to Dr. Charles H. Hillman and colleagues (2006) at the University of Illinois at Urbana. The researchers, who focused primarily on aerobic exercise, found that fitness appears to improve executive function in school-aged children. Students who exercised had higher math and reading scores on standardized tests (Hillman et al., 2008). Findings by Pontifex, Saliba, Raine, Picchietti, and Hillman in 2013 demonstrated similar benefits for children with ADHD. Yoga has also been shown to improve executive function more effectively than simple stretching and strengthening exercise among older adults (Gothe et al., 2014). In a study with college students comparing yoga to aerobic exercise, the yoga group improved significantly in executive function, "contra-dicting some of the previous findings in the acute aerobic exercise and cognition literature" (Gothe et al., 2013, p. 488; see Chapter 13 for more on yoga and executive function).

In 2010, NIH nurse researchers Alyson Ross and Sue Thomas conducted a review of studies comparing the health benefits of yoga and aerobic exercise. Their findings were significant for yoga as an exercise intervention: "Yoga may be as effective as or better than exercise at improving a variety of health-related outcome measures . . . in both healthy and diseased populations (Ross & Thomas, 2010, p. 3).

Children have demonstrated improvements in fitness as a result of school yoga. In a Los Angeles school where the Yoga Ed. curriculum was implemented for one year, fifth graders scored 23.4% higher and seventh graders 28.5% higher than controls in state fitness tests (Slovacek et al., 2003).

Yoga for Fitness

Yoga serves an important role in getting children moving. Its benefits parallel or exceed those of many other forms of exercise, with elements to improve strength, flexibility, balance, and sensory processing.

STRENGTH

Yoga builds strong bodies, strong minds, and a stronger sense of self. Most people think of yoga as a means to increase flexibility. But yoga also builds strong bones (Sparrowe & Walden, 2004) and strengthens joints (Fishman & Saltonstall, 2008). Through stress relief, yoga fortifies the immune system, increasing stamina and the ability to fend off illness. The diaphragm, the muscle of respiration, is strengthened by deep breathing (Cleveland Clinic Foundation, 2014).

In yoga, students use their own body weight to strengthen muscles used in standing and balancing postures. Muscles work in a number of ways in yoga postures. Concentric contraction results in movement, as in dynamic postures; isometric contraction builds strength and stability while holding postures, with-out movement. Both forms of contraction can be combined in Tall Tree, which can be done as a moving flow (concentric) or by holding in the pose (isometric;

see Part V, Unit 3). Eccentric contraction—stretching a muscle while it is working—is especially strengthening. An example is the upward movement in seated Folded Leaf. When coming up with a straight spine—in the strength variation—the abdominal muscles maintain their contraction while they are lengthening throughout the ascent. In addition to working the back muscles concentrically, this requires the muscles in the front of the body to work eccentrically. By learning to identify and contract muscles that are needed to perform new positions, children build new pathways within the brain (Doidge, 2007). In so doing, they gain a sense of mastery and confidence in their own bodies. This can also strengthen their commitment to fitness.

Many yoga postures strengthen the large muscles in the back of the body, making it easier for children to sit and stand up straight. When children sit up straighter in class, their respiration is deeper and they are likely to be more alert. With stronger postural muscles, they can hold themselves erect, affecting how teachers and classmates perceive them.

Feeling strong makes it easier for children to stand upright, to walk with greater ease, and to stand up for themselves. Research shows that an erect posture makes one a less likely victim of harassment (Book et al., 2013). For a strengthening lesson, see Part V, Unit 3.

FLEXIBILITY

You probably remember Aesop's fable about the oak tree and the reed. The oak boasted of her strength and belittled the reed for its weakness in yielding to the wind. When the wind intensified and grew fierce, it yanked the oak out of the ground by its roots. The flexible reed, though bent and flattened, remained, unbroken by the wind.

Just like Aesop's lesson, the key to flexibility is lack of resistance in a posture—no strain, no bouncing, no interruption to the breathing. This is exactly what yoga teaches. Comfortably holding a position increases flex-

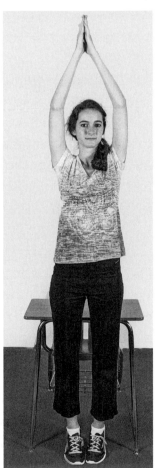

11-1   Tall Tree

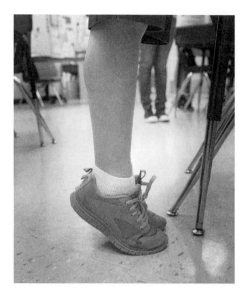

11-2   Contracted Calf

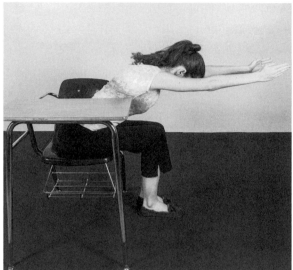

11-3   Folded Leaf Strength

ibility, whereas forcing a stretch tightens the muscle. When we force a stretch, a protective mechanism called the stretch reflex contracts the muscle to prevent injury (Coulter, 2001). Gentle stretching, however, allows the Golgi tendon organ that controls this reflex to "relax . . . and reset the muscle . . . tension" (Robin 2009). The longer the hold, the greater the release; stretching helps individuals feel less "uptight" (Robin, 2009, pp. 449–450). Flexibility can also be increased by repetitive movements—stretching and releasing for brief intervals.

There should be no pain in a yoga practice. Characteristic of all yoga poses, remember, is a comfortable, steady posture (Feuerstein, 1998). Helping a child find comfort in a yoga pose may require simplifying and adapting positions. Watch that students aren't holding their breath or comparing themselves to others. Like the oak and the reed, it is natural for people to respond to movement in different ways.

Remind students about the reed, who yielded to the wind and prevailed. With steady practice, their bodies will likely become more agile and their comfort in posture will increase. By stretching and releasing muscular tension, they will experience a greater openness in their bodies. A less rigid body contributes to greater flexibility in dealing with others, a more relaxed outlook, an increased ease in being. For a brief lesson in flexibility, see Unit 3.

BALANCE AND SENSORY INTEGRATION

Yoga is an exercise regimen that brings balance into the body. Unlike most sports or other forms of exercise, every movement is performed equally on both sides of the body. The varied postures move the spine in all directions, with forward bending, back bending, side bending, and rotation. Through stretching and strengthening muscles, yoga promotes greater comfort and ease in walking, sitting, and standing still.

The endocrine and the nervous systems work together to maintain homeostasis—a balanced state within the body. Slow steady respiration, forward bending, and gentle stretching help slow the nervous system, regulating the flow of blood to the endocrine system (Weintraub, 2012) and enhancing the reabsorption of stress hormones (Cole, 2007). While calming postures promote parasympathetic dominance of the nervous system, energizing postures trigger the sympathetic response (McCall, 2007). Switching between energizing and calming postures, as we do in yoga, facilitates a deeper experience of relaxation of body and mind.

In addition to bringing overall balance to the body, yoga strengthens important neural pathways and sensory systems that orient the body relative to its position in space—proprioception. Sensory integration, the ability of the brain to receive, organize, and use sensory input, affects how an individual perceives his body and his surroundings, his capacity to learn new skills and develop adaptive behaviors, and how he moves, thinks, acts, feels, and relates to others (Ayres, 1995; Kranowitz, 2005).

Vestibular Function

The vestibular system detects movement, balance, and the position of the body, important aspects of sensory processing. The vestibular apparatus consists of receptors for equilibrium, located in the inner ear. These tiny organs help us maintain our balance by motions of the eyes and head and by activating postural reflexes throughout the body (Coulter, 2001). The vestibular system affects the sense of equilibrium, muscle tone, vision, and hearing, as well as emotional security (Kranowitz, 2005).

The visual sense is also part of the vestibular system, which explains why using the eyes to focus on a spot on the floor improves balance. There is evidence that balance postures may be helpful to children who have deficits in the visual-motor channel (Robin, 2009) and that balance and eye-tracking exercises can improve reading skills among children with dyslexia (Young, 2001).

Bilateral Coordination

Bilateral movements are performed by using both sides of the body. Bringing the palms together or crossing the arms or one foot over the other—movements used in Tree balances and Eagle pose—are examples. Bilateral movements have been shown to enhance the growth of new brain cells in stroke victims (Cauraugh & Summers, 2005) and to improve gross and fine motor coordination. These motions enhance sensory processing skills and impact brain development.

When I was in high school, I worked with a group of volunteers to assist a child with severe brain damage. Together, we moved the child's limbs to simulate swimming and crawling motions to enhance communication skills and muscle coordination. These movements are believed to improve communication between

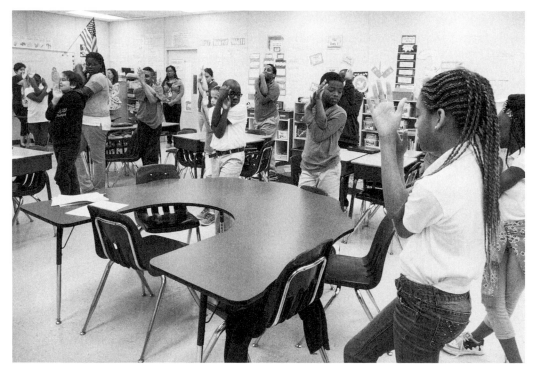

11-4   Eagle Pose

the two hemispheres of the brain. Brain Gym, long used in classrooms, is a system of simple exercises originating from "ancient disciplines such as yoga," designed to enhance "whole brain learning through movement repatterning" (Dennison & Dennison, 1986, pp. i–ii). Like Brain Gym, yoga breaks incorporate bilateral movements in many postures that cross the midline of the body and help wake up the brain.

Cerebellum

The job of the cerebellum, located at the back of the brain, is to maintain equilibrium and correct posture. Neuropsychiatrist John Ratey calls the cerebellum the "rhythm and blues" center of the brain because "this center also coordinates thoughts, attention, emotions, and even social skills. . . . When we exercise, particularly if the exercise requires complex motor movements, we're also exercising the areas of the brain involved in the full suite of cognitive functions" (Ratey, 2008, p. 41). Yoga balance postures help activate the networks that solidify these connections within the brain (Ratey, 2008).

Balance and Focus

Yoga requires a balance of effort and effortlessness. The practice of standing with one foot off the ground strengthens muscles and joints, but it also requires flexibility. A rigid body cannot make those tiny adjustments and subtle shifts needed to hold a balance pose. "Yoga involves the equal exertion of all parts of the body and does not overstrain any one part" (Iyengar, 2001, p. 19).

In addition to improving vestibular function and bilateral coordination, balance poses demand the student's full attention. Balance poses are an excellent practice in paying attention.

Iyengar yoga teacher and scientist Roger Cole (2007) explains, "The instant we lose focus, we fall over. . . . Standing on one foot, we naturally drop extraneous thoughts to focus on the task at hand. That's why these poses . . . require intense, unwavering alertness. . . . The sustained effort to center and recenter, when successful, brings not only our flesh and bones into balance but also our nerve impulses, thoughts, emotions, and very consciousness. Hence, we feel calm. Equilibrium brings equanimity," which, in turn, allows for greater focus. There are balance exercises throughout the BREATHE FIRST curriculum. For a balance routine, see Unit 3.

Educators agree that getting young people moving is important. Opportunities to take even a short movement break during their day can enhance learning. Research has demonstrated numerous health and academic benefits to schoolchildren who are physically fit. Studies suggest that yoga is as good as or better than aerobic exercise for improving essential skills for scholastic success. Yoga is a fitness program that builds strength and flexibility, as well as improving balance and sensory processing skills.

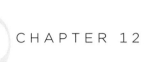

CHAPTER 12

Yoga Promotes Self-Regulation and Resilience

S ELF-REGULATION AND SELF-CONTROL are tools for navigating the inevitable stresses that accompany learning and growing. Resilience is the quality that enables individuals to overcome extraordinary challenges and chart their own course.

Much of the body's response to stress is automatic, as we've seen in Chapter 10. The autonomic nervous system regulates bodily functions that activate and rebalance functions necessary for survival. A great deal of regulation also comes from outside the body. Parents and caregivers respond to a child's need for food, shelter, reassurance, and love. When this happens in a predictable manner, most children learn to anticipate that they will get what they need (Perry, 2015). This is the first step in making short-term stress more tolerable.

The community around the child also affects patterns of regulation. A chaotic existence triggers increased stress responses; a stable environment helps the nervous system retain homeostasis. Educators provide structure in school with guidelines for learning, behavior, and safety. Consistent encouragement and outcomes promote further tools to regulate a youth's emotional development.

Part of the process of maturing requires active participation in one's own regulation—learning to "tolerate the sensations of distress that accompany an unmet need" (Perry, 2015). Self-regulation is a form of self-control. Although the terms are often used interchangeably, there is a difference. Self-regulation implies a deep bodily response, an internal shift from sympathetic to parasympathetic dominance of the autonomic nervous system—from stress to balance. There is an emotional component to self-regulation; it changes how a person feels.

Self-control is a form of regulation characterized by will. A person can control his actions by sheer force of will without resetting his emotions. Self-control implies restraint, which is a behavioral response. Self-control can be an important aspect of self-regulation. Changing one's behavior often precedes a positive emotional adjustment.

In this chapter, we examine the power of self-control, self-regulation, and resilience, and explore how yoga breaks enhance these skills.

The Case for Self-Control

Any teacher can verify that self-control is a factor in scholastic and social success. A longitudinal study of 164 eighth grade students demonstrated its importance as twice that of IQ (Duckworth & Seligman, 2005). Research by Tangney, Baumeister, and Boone (2004) noted the relationship between self-control and elevated self-esteem, better social skills, and fewer incidents of alcohol abuse and binge eating among adolescents.

Terrie Moffitt and colleagues expanded this view after following over 1,000 children from Dunedin, New Zealand, from birth through age 32. Researchers found that children who exhibited better self-control were more likely to become healthy, independent, financially solvent adults, and that improving self-control at any stage resulted in better outcomes. "Interventions addressing self-control might reduce a panoply of societal costs, save taxpayers money, and promote prosperity" (Moffitt et al., 2011, p. 2693).

Yoga and Self-Regulation

In an exploration of yoga as a tool for self-regulation, a research team led by Dr. Tim Gard of Massachusetts General Hospital considered the self-regulatory components of yoga. "There is emerging evidence from the extant literature . . . that modern adaptations of yoga practice are beneficial for mental and physical health . . . facilitating self-regulation and resulting in psychological and physical well-being" (Gard, Noggle, et al., 2014, p. 14). The researchers speculate that through regular yoga practice, the process of "self-regulation [will] become more automatized and efficient over time, requiring less effort to initiate when necessary and terminate more rapidly when no longer needed" (p. 1).

In social interactions fraught with tension, students often respond reflexively based upon past experiences. Regular yoga breaks give many students an opportunity to reframe their perception of an offense, and to adjust their response. In previous chapters we've heard examples of less bullying, fewer suspensions, and improved social interaction among students who have practiced yoga.

Jennifer Frank, assistant professor at Penn State University, is codeveloper of Transformative Life Skills. This secular yoga-based program promotes social-emotional wellness for adolescents in middle and high school in 15-, 30-, or 60-minute lessons. Research gleaned from the program suggests a decrease in hostility among participants: "We are finding significant and meaningful effects on measures of student engagement in school, emotion regulation, mental health and precursors to violence among students in high-risk inner-city communities" (personal communication, April 9, 2015).

Many of the students I work with use yoga skills to help them redirect anger. A second grader shared his use of Shake It Out to restrain his tendency to throw things when he gets frustrated playing video games. "I just jump up and shake my whole body instead!"

Breathing techniques help many young people regain control. A Pennsylvania physical education teacher described a student who used to fight continually with her sister. After practicing yoga in her PE classes, she began to substitute three-part breathing (see Unit 3) instead of responding with her fists (personal communication, August 19, 2014).

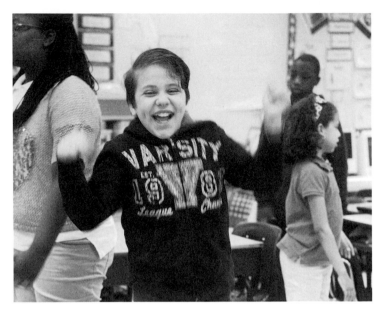

12-1   Shake It Out

Stefanie Gross coaches her high school students to use their guided relaxation session at the end of their Move through Yoga classes to "push the reset button." One of her students told me:

> I've always had anger issues. I've been suspended so many times; been in a lot of trouble. When I switched into yoga, I was skeptical. There were all these positions to learn. But my teacher smiles a lot. The class is welcoming. I started doing stretches. Now I [participate] in every class.
>
> My mother keeps asking me, "What's different about you? What's changing?" She can tell that I'm not so angry anymore, and she can't figure out why. (personal communication, January 27, 2015)

Robert Sapolsky notes the connection between anxiety, fear, and aggressive behaviors: "Anxiety seems to wreak havoc in the limbic system, the brain region concerned with emotion. . . . The amygdala, which is involved in the perception of and response to fear-evoking stimuli . . . is also central to aggression, underlying the fact that aggression can be rooted in fear" (2003, p. 88).

Research has shown significant decreases in gray matter density in the amygdala (the part of the brain that processes fear) after an 8-week mindfulness program including sitting meditation and yoga (Hölzel et al., 2010). A later study by these scientists revealed increases in gray matter density in other areas of the brain related to regulation and learning. The "results suggest that participation in [Mindfulness-Based Stress Reduction] is associated with changes in gray matter concentration in brain regions involved in learning and memory processes, emotion regulation, self-referential processing, and perspective taking" (Hölzel et al., 2011, p. 36).

In 2010, researcher Tamar Mendelson and colleagues examined the effectiveness of a yoga and mindfulness program for 97 fourth and fifth graders in the Baltimore public schools. Developed and taught by the Holistic Life Foundation, the 12-week program for at-risk youth included postures, breathing, and mindfulness relaxation. The researchers concluded that yoga is an effective intervention for alleviating stress and improving self-regulation, particularly in the areas of "rumination, intrusive thoughts, and emotional arousal" (Mendelson et al., 2010, p. 985). "Enhancing regulatory capacities . . . among at-risk youth has the potential to facilitate development of core competencies that will promote a range of positive emotional, behavioral, and academic outcomes" (p. 992).

Emotional Regulation

Katherine Ghannam is the founder of Headstand, a San Francisco–based school yoga program. In addition to movement, units revolve around social-emotional content such as compassion and kindness. Students sit together in

> restorative circles to address problems in class and to identify their feelings through talking, journaling, breathing, and meditation.
>
> Throughout the class, the teacher asks, "How're you feeling?" There's call and response, quick answers while they're holding a pose. We help them understand changes to their physical and emotional state through yoga; how crazy our minds can be. That meditation can be frustrating; it's not going to bring about immediate calm. Sometimes other emotions need to surface first—anger and frustration. (personal communication, January 22, 2015)

The purpose of yoga is not to remove strong emotions. Rather, it helps young people make an inner connection, to acknowledge their feelings and to learn that these feelings do not define who they are. Through the process of experiencing, sharing, and addressing their emotions, students increase their capacity to self-regulate.

Cheryl Crawford was an Atlanta classroom teacher and longtime YogaKids trainer before cofounding Grounded Yoga.

Many high school kids feel angry and scared. They have a right to that feeling. It's not enough to tell them to think positive thoughts. They need to work on their anger, do something with it. There's a lot of fire in them. That's great energy! We ask, "What can you do with this fiery energy?"

We start with strength poses. Then breathing. The kids journal every day—at first many say they don't feel anything. They're numb. Then gradually, they're able to notice their feelings. Slowly they begin to connect the feelings in their body with their emotions. We had a student who had lost his brother. We allowed him to feel his sadness. He took that sad feeling and created a personal yoga flow—a sweet, purposeful, watery flow. He learned what worked for him—something he could use any time to process his feelings of loss. (personal communication, March 13, 2015)

Body Image and Self-Regulation

Young people often feel at odds with their bodies, especially during adolescence, when changes are rapid and unpredictable. During the period in their lives when they are most susceptible to peer pressure and self-doubt, young people are bombarded with media images that portray a physical ideal that rarely matches what they see in the mirror. No matter how beautiful they may appear to us, they see themselves as too tall or too fat; their hair is too straight or too curly. Their noses are too long or too short. This disdain sometimes results in dangerous choices.

In a 2006 study, Scime and colleagues examined the impact of a prevention program for eating disorders combining yoga, discussion, and relaxation. The program, involving 45 fifth grade girls over a 10-week period, "resulted in a significant decrease on scales measuring body dissatisfaction and drive for thinness, as well as media influence" (Scime et al., 2006, p. 143).

One of the researchers in the study, psychologist Catherine Cook-Cottone, is associate professor at the State University of New York at Buffalo and founder of

Yogis In Service. She points to research suggesting that even very young children can learn and effectively practice self-regulation techniques to change body awareness (Cook-Cottone, 2015; Merritt et al., 2012).

In her program, Cook-Cottone combines known eating disorder preventive techniques with yoga "to help young girls develop an effective and positive sense of self. Over the past 10 years we have found this program to reduce body dissatisfaction and drive for thinness as well as increase active self-care practices" (personal communication, August 25, 2015).

Cook-Cottone makes the case for prevention through changing a child's relationship with her body: "Children appear to benefit from the concrete, embodied components of prevention programs that address self-regulation and self-care (e.g., active yoga practice, relaxation strategies, feeling identification and coping). . . . To recover, or *avoid illness in the first place*, individuals must learn to be with, and in, their bodies in a healthy and effective way" (2016, p. 99).

Resilience

Resilience is the ability to adapt to and rebound from high levels of stress. Research shows that the more trauma an individual is exposed to, especially in childhood, the more rapidly his nervous system moves into stress mode. Adversity in early childhood has long been associated with lower school achievement (Tyrka et al., 2013), chronic illness, and interpersonal challenges (CDC, 2015a). In an effort to explain why some children succeed despite such extreme hardships, a 2015 report from the Center on the Developing Child at Harvard University (2015b) examined the essence of resilience.

The report cited four "counterbalancing factors" that contribute to resilience in children: the presence of a caring, supportive parent or caregiver (or teacher, counselor, or coach); helping children develop an experience of mastery over their own lives; developing strong executive function and self-regulation skills; and a solid tradition based on faith or culture. When children believe that they are capable of charting their own course and they are supported in that process, they are more likely to tolerate adversity than others in comparable circumstances—to turn "toxic stress" to "tolerable stress" (Center on the Developing Child at Harvard University, 2015b, p. 4).

As discussed in Chapter 10, sustained periods of acute stress may diminish the growth of brain cells and brain connections, shrinking the hippocampus (Gage, 2003). It is in this area of the limbic system that information is organized and stored. Once the stress has passed, the hippocampus is capable of regaining its original size; long-lasting trauma, however, has been shown to interfere with the recovery process (Bremner et al., 2000), increasing the risk of diminished reserves—mentally, physically, and emotionally.

Activities that strengthen the overall health of children, such as physical exercise and meditation, enhance their ability to recover from extreme stress (Center on the Developing Child at Harvard University, 2015b). The report encourages schools to provide opportunities "for meaningful participation and belonging, as well as for the development of . . . cognitive skills and self-regulation abilities" (p. 9).

Opportunities for Mastery

Sarah is a high school student on the autism spectrum who has taken my Creative Relaxation yoga classes since middle school. She is a lovely young lady, with an amazing memory for detail and a wonderful sense of humor. The challenge for her is to contain her excitement, which sometimes triggers rocking or hand flapping behaviors. In yoga classes, we alternate playful postures that promote social interactions with calming poses that promote regulation. In this way students can have fun with their peers without becoming overwhelmed by excessive stimulation. When Sarah's enthusiasm starts to overtake her, I cue her to breathe or hug her knees, postures that evoke a calming effect.

Sarah's mother told me that her daughter's face lights up whenever she talks about yoga.

It makes her happy! Like so many people with autism, she loves the routine of yoga. She looks forward to going to class. It's so difficult for children with autism to socialize; this provides an outlet to socialize in a small setting, around people she feels safe with—where she has friends.

I think for Sarah, more than anything else, it gives her confidence. Invaluable confidence! She gets a sense of accomplishment doing the postures. Being with friends helps with her self-esteem. It's about so much more than the postures (personal communication, August 7, 2015)

Young people of diverse backgrounds have demonstrated improvements in academic performance, fitness, self-esteem, and conduct as a result of school yoga programs. After a year of Yoga Ed. with 405 students, grades K–8, in an inner-city school, "Yoga and discipline referrals were negatively correlated, with higher participation in yoga related to higher grade point averages. The study reported a 20% increase in students' self-esteem after completing the Yoga Ed. program," according to Brynne Caleda, CEO (personal communication, April 1, 2015; Slovacek et al., 2003).

These outcomes are encouraging when considering the role of yoga in enhancing self-regulation and resilience relative to school performance.

Mastery and Prevention: Breaking the School-to-Prison Pipeline

Carla Barrett is assistant professor of sociology at John Jay College of Criminal Justice in New York. She conducted a 9-month qualitative study on an alternative to incarceration program for 16–24-year-olds who were permitted to serve their sentences in a special school rather than jail. The program included yoga and meditation through the Lineage Project as well as anger management, behavior and group therapy, mental health assessment, and drug prevention counseling. Attendance and progress were monitored by a case worker who reported periodically to the presiding judge; if students were not in compliance, they went directly to jail.

The biggest surprise in interviewing these students was how many young men told stories of incidents on the street where they would normally have gotten into a fight, which would have meant getting kicked out of the program. They were able to de-escalate because of what they learned in yoga. One youth told me, "Without even thinking about it, I just started doing my yoga breathing." The response came to their bodies first before it came to their minds. Another said, "I didn't even realize it. I just started taking deep breaths and my body calmed down."

Yoga is complementary to anger management programs. Some students said, "They tell us not to be angry, but I have a lot to be angry about. In yoga they tell us to take deep breaths. That works."

There are extremely high rates of trauma among court-involved youth, from direct sexual assault to witnessing violence in their communities. We are not talking enough about the role of trauma in the school-to-prison pipeline. The Lineage Project is dealing with stress as well as emotional regulation challenges. It's not just a yoga class; the teachers include movement, meditation, and discussion about the challenges of being locked up and other problems that these young people have.

From the research I do in general, the cost effectiveness of rehab programs reflect an amazing return on the investment. It costs over $200,000 a year to lock up one kid. If they go to upstate detention, there's an 80% recidivism rate. Prevention—positive interventions and alternative programs—reduces recidivism. To bring a yoga program like Lineage into a suspension school is a great investment. If we spend that money now to teach self-regulation skills, we may keep young people from ending up in juvenile court later. (Carla Barrett, personal communication, October 8, 2014)

Through self-control and self-regulation, students develop the ability to cope with, adapt to, and learn from stressful episodes. This is resilience. It is this characteristic that permits young people to overcome extraordinary obstacles and redirect the course of their lives. Chapters 16 and 17 offer specific yoga breaks for enhancing these skills.

CHAPTER 13

Executive Function

SUCCESSFUL STUDENTS HAVE the ability to focus, shift their attention, and stay on task. These aspects of executive function have a tremendous impact on an individual's capacity to learn. In many cases, these factors, along with resilience, self-regulation, and the ability to manage stress exceed the influence of raw intelligence.

The Center on the Developing Child (2011) at Harvard University compares the ability to focus, assess distractions, and shift gears to an air traffic control center. Just as the air traffic center at a busy airport monitors countless incoming and outgoing flights at multiple terminals, the brain's executive function manages the multiple demands simultaneously made upon us.

Three types of brain function regulate executive function (Center on the Developing Child, 2015a):

- "Working memory governs our ability to retain and manipulate distinct pieces of information over short periods of time.

- Mental flexibility helps us to sustain or shift attention in response to different demands or to apply different rules in different settings.
- Self-control enables us to set priorities and resist impulsive actions or responses."

We discussed self-control in Chapter 12; now we'll concentrate on the other characteristics of executive function.

Working Memory

Memory, both long and short term, is the domain of the hippocampus, part of the limbic system (Kumaran, 2008), which has the capacity to increase in size (neurogenesis) during periods of peak learning (Maguire et al., 2000). Exercise and stimulation have also been shown to trigger brain cell growth (Gage, 2003) and improve memory (Holloway, 2003).

Students' emotional state at the time of instruction influences their capacity to retain instruction. When learning is a positive, pleasurable experience, dopamine facilitates the processing of information from brain cell to brain cell. If a child is stressed or anxious, his memory is not receptive to storing new information (Willis, 2008). The hippocampus actually shrinks during prolonged periods of stress (Gage, 2003) or depression (Vythilingam et al., 2002), which may explain why learning is especially challenging for children who live in chronic fear or deprivation.

Both working memory and mental flexibility require the ability to control and shift attention. Fluid intelligence is the ability to cope with "novel environments and . . . abstract reasoning" (Sternberg, 2008, p. 6791). Research demonstrates that fluid intelligence can be increased through working memory, a process that uses neural networks similar to working memory and that also requires control of attention (Jaeggi et al., 2008). These processes, essential to learning, generally decline with age.

In a 2014 study with older adults, Gard, Taquet, and colleagues discovered that the "age-related decline in fluid intelligence is slower in yoga practitioners and meditators" than in carefully matched controls (p. 7). They also found that "yoga practitioners have more resilient networks than controls and meditators"

(p. 5) and that "mindfulness . . . was positively correlated with fluid intelligence and global brain network efficiency and resilience" (p. 10).

A 2013 study examined the effects of yoga versus aerobic exercise on executive function among college-aged women. "Results showed that cognitive performance after the yoga exercise . . . was significantly superior (i.e., shorter reaction times, increased accuracy) as compared with the aerobic and baseline conditions for both inhibition and working memory tasks" (Gothe et al., 2013, p. 488).

These findings provide incentive for implementing yoga and mindfulness breaks to enhance executive function among youth.

Mental Flexibility

Flexibility and attention are the purview of yoga. Most any yoga teacher will make the case that a flexible body is the first step toward a more flexible mind.

According to ancient literature, yoga practices were originally designed to prepare the body to sit in stillness (Feuerstein, 1998). Physical pain is considered an obstacle to this end. A rigid, inflexible body cannot sit or move comfortably in any position. By creating space in joints and length in muscles, yoga helps children regain a freedom within the body and mitigates some of the distractions from physical discomfort.

Learning is enhanced by feeling calm. Yoga is a widely acknowledged form of stress reduction. Gothe and colleagues (2013) point out that feelings of relaxation and calm, a frequent aftereffect of yoga, may contribute to such qualities as self-control and concentration. Whereas "lowered mood is associated with declines in cognitive function" (Gothe et al., 2013, p. 493), yoga is an intervention that has been shown to elevate mood and reduce stress (Conboy et al., 2013; Mendelson et al., 2010; Streeter et al., 2010) and enhance cognition (Birdee et al., 2009; Rocha et al., 2012).

What distinguishes yoga from most other forms of exercise is the mental focus that accompanies both exercise and stillness. Movements of the body are in concert with the activity of the mind. The Gothe study notes the correlation between improved focus and executive function: "The practice of yoga emphasizes body awareness and involves focusing one's attention on breathing or specific muscles or parts of the body; therefore it is possible that yoga may improve more general attentional abilities. Attentional focus is a major aspect of yoga practice" (Gothe et al., 2013, p. 494).

Improved attention correlates to improved school performance. In a 2014 study of 49 adolescents in an urban inner-city school district, Frank and colleagues examined the effectiveness of Transformative Life Skills. "Although the mechanisms of action are not fully understood, it appears that yoga and meditative practices evoke a calming effect, which helps students get into a frame of mind conducive to learning and distinctive from the effects of physical exercise alone. The beneficial effects of these practices have been demonstrated among students from a wide variety of backgrounds" (Frank et al., 2014, p. 34).

Before beginning her Mindful Movement program at a Brooklyn high school, teacher Marissa Lipovsky began implementing yoga breathing and movement in her math classes. She experimented by having students try a math problem at the beginning of class; then she would take a short yoga break and give a different problem with similar properties. Lipovsky discovered that yoga "helped rewire their brains and seemed to regulate their thinking. One student used to mix up coordinates in graphing. After the yoga activity, he'd get it right" (personal communication, February 25, 2015).

Sustained Attention

Executive function, according to Daniel Goleman, is the "power to direct our focus onto one thing and ignore others. . . . [This] holds the key to self-management" (2013, p. 77). As yoga teaches, a focused mind is a steady mind.

There has long been compelling evidence among researchers for training the mind to focus fully on one thing at one time. In 1998, Kilgard and Merzenrich discovered that the formation of new pathways in the brain, what we would call learning, requires sustained attention (Doidge, 2007). Not surprisingly, multitasking, a skill so prized in today's culture, is also a deterrent to retaining information. "While you can learn when you divide your attention, divided attention doesn't lead to abiding changes in your brain map" (Doidge, 2007, p. 68).

Teaching students to concentrate on individual areas of the body facilitates their capacity to attend to one thing at one time. The 31-Points Relaxation (Rama, 1982) is a mindful practice for body scanning, point by point. With per-

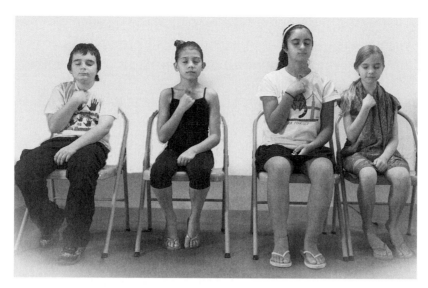

13-1   Focusing Practice

mission from the Himalayan Institute, I've modified this technique for use while seated in classrooms. The teacher leads students through a designated sequence of body points, beginning at the forehead. Students lightly touch each of the 31 places on their upper body with one fingertip. The routine helps students focus their attention as they connect to their own bodies. You'll find this focusing practice in Unit 4.

Balance poses are another excellent method for teaching focus. It's extremely difficult to stand on one foot without the synchrony of breath, mind, and body. Progressive muscle relaxation exercises like Tense and Relax and Floating on a Cloud (see Unit 2) are also tools for improving focus. Taking a student through a guided tour of her body and mind invites her full attention and imagination. By providing a specific point of focus, yoga helps a child rein in her wandering mind. You'll find many focusing exercises throughout the BREATHE FIRST curriculum.

Yoga Breaks to Increase Focus

It's not necessary to be a yoga teacher to implement short yoga breaks to increase focus in a classroom. Sondra Sellitti, a Florida high school English teacher with little yoga experience, graciously participated in an experiment with me. I provided her with a 5-minute yoga break. Using the written instructions that you will find in Unit 2, she implemented the routine at the beginning of class for two groups of high school seniors. Participation was encouraged but not required. After a month of daily practice, she reported the experience a success:

> The exercises were very simple to do. In general, the students enjoyed the stretches and said they "felt better." The students seemed more alert and focused on their work after. Only two or three students of approximately 20–25 in each class declined to participate at all.
>
> I don't have empirical evidence; however, I believe the exercises not only focused students on academics, but they calmed students who have difficulty controlling their behavior to conform with classroom rules and attend to instructions. . . . On a personal note, my neck muscles felt more relaxed, and tension was relieved. It lightened the mood for everyone.

When asked by Sellitti to anonymously report their responses to the yoga breaks, nearly 75% of students responded favorably. Typical comments included:

> "The stretches helped me to release a little bit of tension before getting started with classwork."
> "It's relaxing, and it helps me concentrate better."
> "Helps me wake up and get in a mood ready for work."
> "Good, but need more."
> "A waste of my dog-gone time."
> "Excellent stress reliever—real quick—real fast."

And of course, one student handed in the response, saying, "Whatever" (shrugs shoulders).

At the conclusion of the month-long experiment, I asked if they would continue the program. Ms. Sellitti replied, "Yes, at the students' request, and mine!" (personal communication, March 6, April 2, April 6, 2015).

Yoga breaks mitigate stress through exercise, breathing, relaxation, and focused stillness. Movement enhances learning readiness and processing skills. Through yoga, young people discover that they have choices in how they respond to stress. Movement, stillness, and breathing practices improve self-regulation skills. Applying these techniques in the face of challenge empowers students, promoting resilience and independence.

PART IV

PRINCIPLES OF CREATIVE RELAXATION YOGA

Creative Relaxation is the program I began over 30 years ago for training educators, therapists, yoga teachers, and parents in the implementation of yoga for children in school. Although much of my focus in yoga education has been for children with autism and varying special needs, Creative Relaxation is suitable for students of all abilities, prekindergarten through college. It adapts yoga exercises for use in public school education and in varied therapeutic settings.

The principles of Creative Relaxation are explored in the next four chapters. They are to create a peaceful space, engage the student, provide tools for success, and foster independence (Goldberg, 2004a). The objectives of Creative Relaxation are to support teachers in creating a classroom experience in which students feel safe, involved in learning, focused, and self-sufficient.

Yoga breaks help mitigate stress, invite connections with others, release frustration, and foster self-regulation skills. In addition, yoga practices build a community where children can laugh, share, and interact with kindness. Creative Relaxation teaches children to reflect and make conscious choices, as well as to befriend and listen to their own bodies.

CHAPTER 14

Create a Peaceful Space

OUR FIRST PRIORITY as educators is to create an environment where every student is free from harm. When working with a classroom of diverse students, teachers do not always know to what extent their students have been touched by trauma. For this reason, creating a peaceful space within the classroom is especially important. Feeling safe provides a respite from a world that can be unkind and even cruel. Opportunities for quiet and introspection empower students to develop resources for dealing with stress, and help them recognize the distinction between chaos and calm. Participating within a benevolent community builds trust and confidence.

Feeling Safe

Fears of abuse, punishment, or rejection rule the lives of many children. According to the Centers for Disease Control and Prevention (CDC, 2016), 702,000 victims of child abuse and neglect were confirmed in 2014. The CDC (2016) estimated that "1 in 4 children experience some form of child maltreatment in their lifetimes," and reported over 1,600 deaths in 2014 from neglect or abuse.

The effects of childhood trauma continue to inform the life of the individual into adulthood. A 2007 study revealed a "very strong association between childhood adversity and depressive symptoms, antisocial behavior, and drug use during the early transition to adulthood. These finding . . . indicate the critical need for prevention and intervention strategies" (Schilling et al., 2007, p. 9).

Audrey Tyrka of Brown University Medical School and colleagues have researched the impact of childhood adversity on endocrine function and immunity, noting links between "childhood adversity [and] . . . medical conditions such as cardiovascular disease and diabetes" (Tyrka et al., 2013, p. 434). In an e-mail conversation, Tyrka acknowledged that providing tools for stress relief could potentially reduce long-term effects of childhood stress, such as the propensity toward illness or depression (personal communication, October 9, 2012).

Tyrka's research suggests that extreme stress due to childhood trauma is "linked to alterations in HPA axis" (Tyrka et al., 2012, p. 7). The HPA axis triggers the influx of stress hormones, slowing digestive, reproductive, and immune function; it is also responsible for shutting off the stress circuit (McEwen, 2002). A compromised HPA axis may explain the tendency among those with a history of extreme childhood stress to be more reactive and less controlled in their response to adversity. Without tools to manage their stress, their nervous systems revert more quickly to fight-or-flight mode.

"Being able to feel safe with other people is probably the single most important aspect of mental health," according to psychiatrist Bessel van der Kolk, who works with trauma survivors in his Boston clinic. "Social support is the most powerful connection against becoming overwhelmed by stress or trauma. . . . For our physiology to calm down, heal, and grow we need a visceral feeling of safety" (2014, p. 79). Van der Kolk implements yoga postures, breathing, and meditation in his work to mitigate the impact of trauma.

Many children don't know how it feels to be safe or how to acknowledge the extent of their anxiety. Yoga breaks provide opportunities for children to acquaint themselves with the sensations within their own bodies. They learn that there are adjustments that they can make through breathing and movement that change how they feel.

One high school senior, a well-regarded athlete in an inner-city school, spoke to me after he had been taking a school yoga class for about 6 months: "One thing that's helped me a lot is the breathing. I'm claustrophobic. When I'm in an elevator, if it's taking too long, I panic. It's a bad feeling. Now I know how to breathe. I just take a deep breath, close my eyes, and it's okay." Just talking about the elevator changed this young man's demeanor from cool to anxious. As he demonstrated his deep breath, I saw tension drain from his face (personal communication, January 27, 2015).

Finding Stillness

Yoga has taught me the importance of taking a minute to be still, listen to my thoughts and relax. (Bobbi, senior, Williamsburg Prep High School, courtesy Anne Desmonde, Bent on Learning, personal communication, January 13, 2015)

If you spend any time in schools, you know how noisy they can be. Hallways are filled with students jostling, hollering, and shrieking. The cafeteria is a roar of continual chatter and shouts; bells squeal; loudspeakers bellow—noise, noise, noise. Silence is enforced during tests and lectures, but there are rarely quiet times during the school day that are not fraught with stress. Outside school, kids are bombarded with loud volumes from TV, computer games, and music.

Research has demonstrated that children exposed to chronic noise during their school day experience higher levels of cortisol and increased stress response, and may function more poorly in school than children in quieter settings (Seidman & Standring, 2010). In fact, "noise significantly elevates stress among children at . . . levels far below those necessary to produce hearing damage" (Evans et al., 1998, p. 75). According to a World Health Organization report, chronic exposure to low-level noise may result in the impairment of cognitive tasks such as "reading, long term memory, attention and motivation" (2009, p. 40).

Quiet has a soothing effect on most mammals, yet it's a "sound" that is unfamiliar to many youth. What happens to children when they are reintroduced to the sound of quiet?

According to Beth Navon, former executive director of Lineage Project in

New York City, young adults crave quiet. The Lineage Project curriculum combines yoga, meditation, and discussion in classes for at-risk and incarcerated youth. Navon notes that many of these young adults, ages 10–24, live in crowded spaces with little opportunity for privacy. "The challenge for many is finding a place in their home or environment where they can be still within their day. Given the chance, their ability to sit quietly knocks me out" (personal communication, August 13, 2014).

With all the fidgeting and finger drumming that accompanies enforced quiet in classrooms, it may be difficult to imagine your students welcoming silence. The Move Through Yoga curriculum includes weekly meditation in their high school classes, starting with 5 minutes and working up to a full 50 minutes of silent sitting. Although it's difficult for many at first, Stefanie Gross says that her students grow to appreciate the quiet. She frequently reminds them, "Silence matters—you have the rest of the day to talk."

> The most beautiful sight for any teacher is seeing her students sitting still. When they leave class after Monday meditation, they say that the world seems louder, more annoying, but also brighter. Observing their peers who scream and gossip, they become aware of the cacophony of unnecessary noise. They tell me, "There's too much stimulation; it's too loud out there." They look forward to their retreat to the yoga room. (Stefanie Gross, personal communication, November 14, 2014)

Importance of Quiet

Stillness gives students an opportunity to reset their inner rhythm. Refocusing attention from outside to inside is the fifth rung of yoga, according to Patanjali. There are many ways to help students turn their attention inward.

In Chime Listening, the teacher strikes a chime one time, instructing students to listen quietly to the sound for as long as possible, then raise their hands when the sound becomes imperceptible (Flynn, 2011). Mindful listening is an excellent tool for quieting a group or to begin a class activity. I often use a singing bowl or vibratone to encourage quiet listening. For more lessons on tuning in, see Part V, Unit 5.

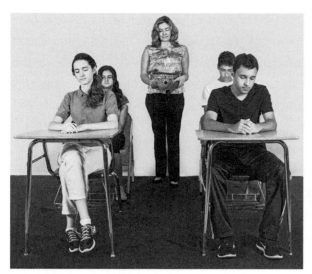

14-1   Setting a Tone

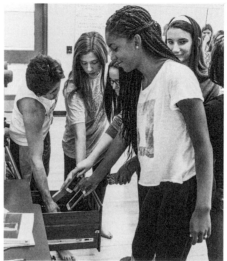

14-2   Tuning Out to Tune In

Donna Davis asks her Edgewater High School PE students to stash their cell phones in her drawer, so they can disconnect from the outside world for 45 minutes each day. Although not required, she highly encourages this commitment to participate fully in class. Yoga, she explains to her students, is about being present and in the moment. Davis sees "many kids addicted to their phones. It's really hard to give it up. When they do it, even for a short time, it's a big thing" (personal communication, April 10, 2015).

Yoga and mindfulness teacher Kelli Love explains that classroom yoga helps students "transfer the emotional regulation strategies that are reinforced daily in the yoga room to everyday school and home environments." The students in her school have a "reflection area in each classroom where they can go to do their own quiet practice if they need a break in their day" (personal communication, December 17, 2014).

Create a Peaceful Mood

Leading your class through a short yoga break at the beginning or end of a lesson is an excellent way to reset the mood. Here's how you might begin.

Dim the lights, put aside your work for a moment, and play soothing music.

If you don't have time to make those adjustments, you can rely on your own voice and breathing to change the tenor of the classroom. These are tools that you have with you at all times. Remember, you are the mirror for your students: They perceive your level of stress or calm. No matter how many times you may tell them to relax or be still, it won't mean much if you are agitated when you say those words.

Breathing in a slow, relaxed manner shifts your body into rest and restore mode. Brown and Gerbarg (2012) recommend "coherent breathing" at approximately six breaths per minute. As your breathing calms, you create an atmosphere of tranquility within your classroom. Using a gentle tone of voice sends a message to your students that you feel safe, that they are safe.

Consciously relax your facial muscles and jaw. Keeping your voice soft, direct your students to take three Huh Breaths (inhaling, shrug the shoulders up to the ears; exhale and drop). Continue with Bellows Breath (see Unit 2): Instruct your students to interlace their fingers and place their hands behind their heads, elbows open. Inhaling, look up; exhaling, look down.

Repeat twice more. Drop the hands and take three more Huh Breaths before returning to normal breathing.

By participating with your students in this 1-minute yoga break, you not only guide them, but you give yourself a moment to relax. In this way you reflect for your students a world that is kind, caring, and calm.

One New Jersey K–8 school uses a 2-minute lesson delivered over the public address system. According to Newark Yoga Movement founder Debby Kaminsky, "Since starting the program two years ago, the principal says that this Monday routine has changed the culture of the school. After a weekend of who knows what, it brings kids back into a place of calm and learning readiness" (personal communication, March 3, 2014).

As difficult as it may be for students to change their thinking or their behavior, it's relatively easy to change how they breathe. Just focusing on the breath creates a calming effect. As the breathing rate slows, the heart rate follows (see Simply Notice, in Unit 4).

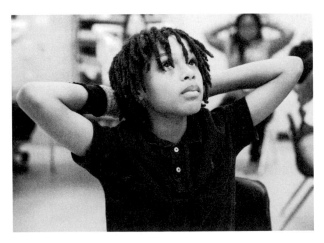

14-3 Bellows Breath Head Rest

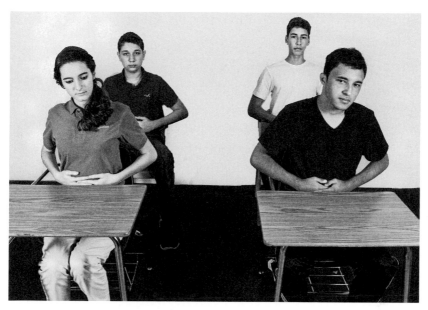

14-4   Soft Belly Breathing

When observing the breath, you may invite students to place their hands on their abdomen. Ask if they notice a gentle movement in this part of their body as they inhale and exhale. Suggest soft belly breathing, in and out through the nose (for instruction, see Unit 1).

Remember, not everyone breathes in the same way. Some may be more aware of their breath in their shoulders or lower ribs (see Follow the Breath under Reset Lessons in Unit 10). Others may be habitual chest breathers. Allergies or asthma makes mouth breathing more natural for some students. It's important to encourage students to breathe in any way that is comfortable for them, to make it a stress-free activity. Simply allowing time for gentle breathing often creates new, more relaxed breathing patterns.

It doesn't take a long time to establish a peaceful mood. Consistent practice is the key. You'll find dozens of calming exercises in the BREATHE FIRST curriculum. The units on breathing, relaxation, and attention are especially useful for creating a peaceful space.

Benevolent Community

By creating a space where students feel safe, where they experience stillness, you transform your classroom into a refuge for your students. This is what

Peace in Schools founder Caverly Morgan calls an "environment of CARE (Confidentiality Acceptance Reverence Empathy)."

Peace in Schools' Mindful Studies is the first semester-long, for-credit high school course offered in the United States, according to Morgan. The pilot program, launched at Wilson High in Portland, Oregon, in 2014, is cotaught by Morgan and yoga educator Allyson Copacino. On the second day of class, students define and create the environment of CARE. Collectively, students agree upon qualities that they will abide by within their classroom. The statement begins, "We agree to maintain an environment that will support mindfulness," and includes words like "compassion, non-judgment, respect, awareness of self and others, teamwork, trust, safety, confidentiality, and honesty." Both Morgan and Copacino have found that when they permit the students to write their own code of behavior and values, these qualities become more than just words.

Copacino explains that through this open and honest interaction, "Teens cultivate trust among their classmates. Establishing an environment of CARE is our way of creating a safe space. Even if students come in anxious, angry, or overwhelmed—whatever they are feeling is accepted and valued here" (personal communication, April 29, 2016).

Making Your Classroom a Peaceful Space

Yoga is a system designed thousands of years ago to help individuals find an experience of peace. The yoga journey, like many classrooms, begins with rules of conduct. Adapted from the *Yoga Sutra* by Patanjali (Feuerstein, 1998), here's what they might look like in your classroom:

Guidelines for Classroom Yoga Breaks

With others:

1. Be kind—Do no harm to others or yourself.
2. Be truthful.
3. Don't mess with others' stuff.
4. Use energy wisely.
5. Take only what you need.

For yourself:

6. Clean up after yourself.
7. Be grateful for what you have.
8. Practice self-discipline.
9. Develop mindful self-awareness.
10. Accept what is.

Throughout the remainder of this book, we will explore methods of implementing these precepts into your classroom through yoga breaks.

CHAPTER 15

Engage the Student

I N CHAPTER 14, we discussed ways to make classrooms peaceful and safe. Those are things that you can do for your students. Engaging children invites their participation in the classroom and school community. Connecting with students is a key step in creating a learning environment.

This became apparent early in my teaching career. As a reading specialist in a Connecticut middle school, I worked with students who were reading well below grade level. Being 13 is tough enough, but for a seventh grader who is reading at a second grade level, it's awful. Many of these children had given up on their own ability to learn; anticipation of failure was well ingrained in them. Others had become class clowns or behavior problems. Acting foolish or rebellious was a good cover for their academic limitations.

Understandably, these students hated to read. Trying to hammer in skills that they had failed at time and time again did not seem a productive approach. Instead, I got to know them and what they cared about. Based on their interests, I chose books or magazines to read to them. They listened; they laughed; they learned. Next they began making up their own stories. If they didn't want to write them, they assigned parts and acted them out. They worked together and talked and shared. We selected one story to expand into a full production—with scenery, costumes, and parts for everyone.

Our reading classroom became a buzz of activity. Students were researching and writing, reading and giggling. Because everyone had a part in the play, students had to develop scripts and learn their lines. They coached and encouraged one another. We invited families and school personnel to the performance, which concluded to thunderous applause. This was something most of these kids had never experienced before.

That year, reading scores soared. Parents called to tell me that their children were feeling better about themselves; they were trying harder with school work; they were engaged in the learning process.

Meeting Students Where They Are

Yoga is uniquely suited to meeting children as and where they are. The brief lessons catch students' interest without overwhelming them. Active students get a chance to get out of their seats and move; if their energy level is low, all they have to do is breathe. Yoga breaks are not graded or evaluated. In every lesson, the teacher sets an example for gentle interaction among students.

Yoga has proven useful for engaging youth in even the most challenging environments. Terri Cooper, founder of The Connection Coalition, formerly Yoga Gangsters, brings yoga to young people in detention centers, where they are understandably cautious about whom they can trust. "Through yoga you make an immediate connection with kids. It's a system that says, 'we are open-minded to who you are and what you are, no matter what you've experienced in your past.' Our motto is 'no blame, no shame, no judgment.'

"After safety, the next most important thing is fun. It's okay to laugh or talk; they're not expected to sit quietly. We don't tell the kids any way they need to change or anything they need to do. We're just there to spend some time together. Through complete acceptance, they begin to open up and connections are created."

Terri shared an exercise that she does with her students to demonstrate the importance of these connections. Standing in one row, arms overlapping, the students step into Warrior 3, a balance pose. Working together, they are sup-

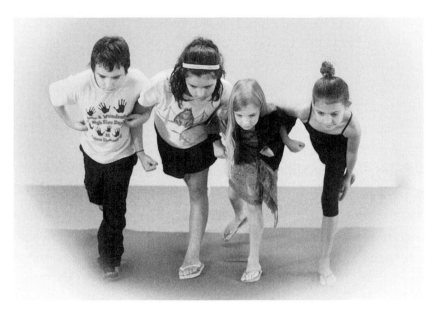

15-1   Group Warrior

ported. If one person drops out, the entire group is destabilized. Cooper uses this to exemplify the importance of the choices and connections these fragile young people make within their community (personal communication, April 21, 2016).

Sleepwalking

Approximately 2,500 years ago, Siddhartha Gautama was born into a privileged life. His protective father isolated him from the world of loss and pain for as long as he could. When he was exposed to the suffering of the outside world, Siddhartha was confused and saddened. He began a quest for understanding, ultimately turning to meditation. It's said that after seven days and seven nights of sitting under a fig tree, he became an illumined teacher. He was known as the Buddha, meaning "enlightened one."

His tranquility drew many people to him. One student asked, "Are you a saint?" The Buddha said no. The student persisted, "Are you a god?" The Buddha said no. Finally the student asked, "What are you?" He replied, "I am awake."

Many of the children in our schools, especially adolescents, seem to be sleep-walking. I have known kids in high school who drift from class to class without interacting with anyone all day long. They say little to their teachers, speak to no one in class, avoid eye contact in the halls, eat lunch alone, and take refuge in the restrooms during breaks—as if to make themselves invisible.

This sense of isolation can contribute to depression and negative self-esteem. The outcome of these behaviors, something that van der Kolk calls "numbing," is a loss of connection to oneself and the inability to "respond . . . to the ordinary demands of the body in quiet, mindful ways." To help patients reconnect with themselves, van der Kolk introduced yoga into his trauma clinic. "Yoga turned out to be a terrific way to gain a relationship with the interior world and with it a caring, loving, sensual relationship to the self" (van der Kolk, 2014, pp. 272–273).

Matthew Sanford (2006) is a world-renowned yoga teacher who specializes in adapting postures for those with physical disabilities. He exudes strength and hope, despite a devastating car accident that paralyzed his lower body. It was this event that forced him to wake up in body and mind. Sanford well under-stands the feeling of being disconnected from his body. He believes that this sense of separation from oneself can contribute to a sense of isolation from others, and may lead to self-destructive behaviors. The practice of yoga can change that: "Each day, as I practice connecting my mind and my body, I am able to feel a more compassionate path" (Sanford, 2008).

One simple yoga exercise that I often use to help students wake up and recon-nect with their bodies is called Tree Breath-ing. Standing up is preferred, but it can also be performed seated. Here's what to do: Starting with the palms pressed together, thumbs at the sternum, inhale and exhale. Notice if the breath causes any movement in the hands—it varies with individuals. With the next inhalation, ele-

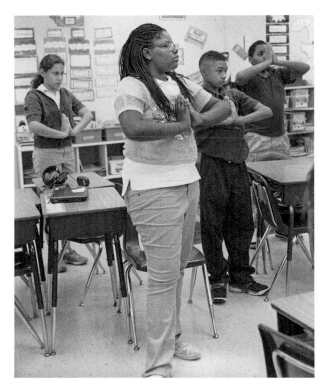

15-2   Tree Breathing

vate the hands overhead, keeping the palms together; lower them with the exhalation. This time watch the hands as they float up with the inhalation and down with the exhalation.

This exercise is beneficial for individuals with impulsivity or attention challenges, who may be unaware of the position of their hands relative to their own or others' bodies. Hand positions such as palms together at the chest help students "collect" themselves. If you notice students' attention drifting, try leading them through a minute or two of Tree Breathing to reengage them before returning to their schoolwork. (You'll find this exercise in Unit 1.)

Making Connections With Others

Much of a student's day, especially in middle or high school, involves listening and receiving information. There may not be much time for genuine give and take, sharing of ideas, or collaboration. Creating an environment where students feel accepted without being judged sets the stage for deeper, more honest connections with others.

Marissa Lipovsky was a math teacher in a Brooklyn high school when she took Bent on Learning yoga teacher training in 2014. Now she is a full-time yoga teacher at the same school; her program is called Mindful Movement. "It's something I never experienced in the math classroom. Knowing they're in a safe place and using mindful listening techniques, students are able to tell their story and be heard. They're really sharing and getting to the root of things they are stressing about. To connect with them and see them letting go—there's a bond formed, not like a regular classroom" (personal communication, February 3 and 25, 2015.

When I followed Yoga 4 Classrooms (Y4C) trainer Sharon Trull through her day at a New Hampshire elementary school, I was impressed by the level of participation among the children. At the beginning of the class, she asked the students to share their preferred methods for finding quiet "alone time," which was the theme for the day. She listened and responded to their comments with encouragement. During the movement portion of class, most students appeared eager to try something new or improve their skills in familiar poses. They welcomed the quiet "desk rest" at the end of the lesson. My favorite part, however, was when each child silently greeted every other student in the room. I watched as children made eye contact, smiled, and acknowledged one another in a genuine way (personal communication, November 25, 2014).

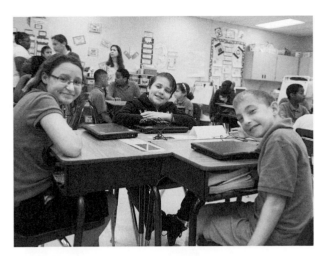

15-3   Greeting Others

It's surprising that kids can spend all day together in school without communicating or learning anything about one another. Because of this, I often begin yoga breaks with the name game (Goldberg, 2013), where the students introduce themselves by first names. Then I challenge the class: "Who can remember everyone's name?"

Once the students know each other, I add variations to the name game. For example, they might begin with their name and their favorite song or band. Another day it might be to name the job of their dreams or their ideal vacation destination—real or imagined. In this brief, stress-free forum, students share a bit of themselves while learning more about their classmates.

My favorite name game is called Something I Like About You. It works well with students seated or standing in a circle. The teacher positions herself next to the child who is the center of attention, so the others will be facing both of them when they share. One student is selected, and everyone says one positive thing about that individual. In a large group, this can be done in written form, signed. Then teachers may highlight one or two students each day by selecting a few statements to be read aloud. It can also be done in smaller groups, with the teacher circulating among them. (You'll find this exercise in Unit 6.)

Clearly, there are parameters. The comments have to be kind, positive, and appropriate for sharing in a group. Students may acknowledge their classmate's personality, physical appearance, clothing, work habits, and so on. Let's say Mark is the student selected. Kids may say that they like his hair or the color of his T-shirt; they think it's awesome that he's such a good guitar player or that he can do an outstanding Warrior pose; they may recall the time that Mark listened to them when they needed someone to talk to.

Every time I've led this game, no matter what his or her classmates choose to say, the student who is the subject of the praise comes away beaming. Sometimes, during the exercise I find myself thinking, "Oh, no, they're only talking about his new shoes and how tall he is." It doesn't matter; every child I've observed is uplifted. It's affirming to be noticed, acknowledged, appreciated in some positive way.

Engaging Through Play

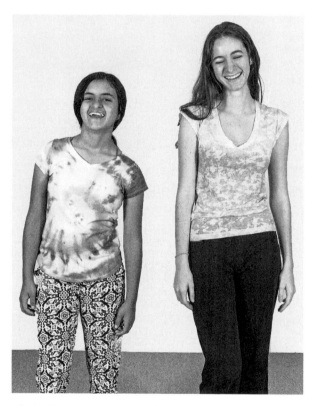

15-4   Engaging Through Play

Research demonstrates the importance of play and social interaction to promote learning. Yet schools offer fewer opportunities for these types of activities. Many schools are now built without playgrounds or gymnasiums for economic reasons. Even recess has been shortened to offer more academic time in many elementary school programs, starting in kindergarten.

Neuroscientist Jaak Panksepp explains that "the urge to play is a neurological drive" and is essential for prompting "positive social engagements and learning" (2007, pp. 58–59). His extensive studies reveal that play enhances social and cognitive development, as well as reducing impulsivity, a characteristic of ADHD. Panksepp's research explains why efforts to subdue extremely active children are often counterproductive: When the urge to play is suppressed, impulsive behaviors and inattention often become more prevalent in classrooms and social interactions. His work demonstrates "that play . . . reduces impulsive behaviors resembling ADHD" and that opportunities for raucous physical play may be therapeutic for those diagnosed with ADHD (Panksepp, 2008, p. 69).

These findings make it especially ironic that the response to students who don't stay on task is often withholding recess.

The forms of unstructured and active play that Panksepp's research finds most beneficial trigger significant changes within the body and the brain. As the heart and respiratory rates accelerate, the brain releases brain-derived neurotrophic factor (BDNF; Ratey, 2008). The protein BDNF is like Miracle-Gro, fertilizer, promoting neurogenesis (the production of new brain cells) and strengthening new connections in the brain (Ratey, 2008). BDNF activates the areas of the brain that enable us to pay attention and retain what we are learning (Doidge, 2007).

Social engagement has a similar effect on brain function. Early researchers discovered that the brains of rodents actually increased in volume and weight in response to stimulation and enriched environments, indicating that new brain cells and connections were being formed (Diamond, Krech, & Rosenzweig, 1964). Studies show that social enrichment among young mice resulted in increased BDNF levels in the adult hippocampus—the part of the brain that retains information. These mice were also more socially interactive and nurturing (Branchi et al., 2006). These studies underscore the importance of play and social engagement in academic and social and emotional learning.

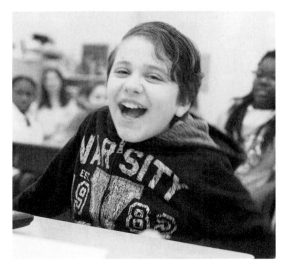

15-5   Having Fun

Having fun is an important balance to the tedium and intensity of the classroom experience for students of all ages. Yoga breaks that combine playful movement and laughter, while no substitute for extended periods of free play, are useful for improving attention and reengaging students.

According to Dr. Lee Berk, associate professor at Loma Linda University, laughter alleviates stress by interrupting the release of cortisol and other stress hormones, while elevating the production of dopamine. Laughter has many of the same benefits as exercise for combating illness, elevating mood, and regulating anxiety (Heid, 2014).

Kidding Around Yoga (KAY) founder Haris Lender incorporates elements of

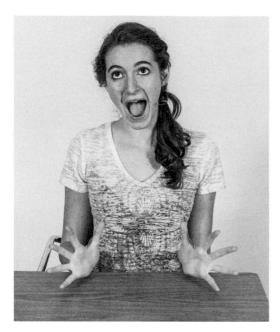

15-6   Lion

Laughter Yoga into her children's yoga program. Developed by Mumbai physician Madan Kataria, Laughter Yoga is an exercise routine combining yoga breathing exercises with laughter without using jokes or even humor. Lender shared one exercise used in the KAY training called Pass-a-Laugh. It starts with students seated in a circle. "The first child turns to his neighbor and lets out a crazy laugh of any kind. That student repeats what he has heard and turns to the next child and lets out a different laugh. That one is also repeated and it goes on and on!" (personal communication, July 6, 2015).

Another yoga pose that induces laughter is also effective for relieving facial tension. I introduce Lion pose as "the prettiest pose in yoga." Here's how it's done: After taking a deep breath, release an exhalation from deep in the belly out the open mouth. Again, take a deep breath in, and this time, stretch the mouth open wide with the exhalation—the tongue reaching down toward the chin, the eyes rolled way up toward the top of the head. Then relax the face and breathe comfortably. When you're ready, take another deep breath. Exhale with a roar from deep in the belly, stretching the face as before. After this huge stretch, relax the face. Once the students are familiar with this posture, they may include the hands, stretching them like claws when they exhale and stretch the face. Although this posture often inspires laughter, it's also an opportunity to release emotional holding from deep within the gut. You'll find Lion pose in Unit 7, and more silly yoga postures in Unit 8.

Imitation

What you say and do around others often has a greater impact than you realize. In 1993, Hatfield and colleagues studied a phenomenon known as "emotional contagion." They found a tendency among individuals to "mimic the facial expressions, vocal expressions, postures, and . . . behaviors of those around them, and . . . to 'catch' others' emotions as a consequence of such facial, vocal, and postural feedback" (Hatfield et al., 1993, p. 97).

Children learn how to interact with others by imitating those around them. This is the initial phase in building deeper connections. In fact, research suggests that it is through imitation that we develop empathy, the capacity to experience another's feelings. That's why the most effective method for teaching children to be kind to one another is by being kind to children and others around us (see Chapter 7).

The process of imitation, according to Marco Iacoboni (2008), is a function of mirror neurons—brain cells that fire when we observe others' facial expressions. Even without understanding the expression on someone's face, our brains respond. Studies using fMRI revealed that while this "inner imitation" is occurring, the mirror neurons send signals to emotional centers that are located in the limbic system within the brain (Iacoboni, 2008, p. 109). This triggers neurons to activate the limbic system. That's when we *experience* the emotions associated with the facial expressions.

Iacoboni explains that mirror neurons help us not only read people, but "feel their suffering" or their joy. Based on this premise, Iacoboni further suggests that good imitators are also good at recognizing emotions; this recognition contributes to a greater capacity to empathize with others. These moments of synchrony with another's feelings, Iacoboni argues, "are the foundation of empathy" (2008, p. 5).

Yoga is a system that is taught through modeling by the teacher and imitation by the student. As the teacher is energized or soothed, she or he mirrors the process of attaining these feelings through movement and breathing.

Empathy: Path to Compassion

Singer, Critchley, and Preuschoff (2009) explored the role of the brain in empathy and decision making. They found that the portion of the brain where we feel our own pain, the anterior insula, is also used to sense others' pain. Singer's work also suggests that both the insula and amygdala are involved in decision making, especially related to intuitive or gut feelings.

In his book *Focus*, Daniel Goleman explains that we use the same network of neurons to glean our own and others' feelings: "The brain's very design seems to integrate self-awareness with empathy. . . . As our mirror neurons and other social circuitry recreate in our brain and body what's going on with the other person, our insula summates all that. Empathy entails an act of self-awareness: we read other people by tuning into ourselves" (2013, p. 104).

In light of this information, we might reconsider our approach to aggressive behaviors such as bullying. It's a common practice to ask children, "How do you think that makes Jacob feel when you say these things?" The student, however, may have no idea how it makes Jacob feel. In order to deepen his ability to understand how someone else feels, we must begin to ask instead, "How do *you* feel?" Bringing awareness to the bodily sensations that accompany specific interpersonal behaviors may be a way for some children to reexamine their choices of words or actions.

In order to increase children's empathy and compassion for their classmates, we need to help them become better observers of their own feelings. This is a process that can be taught through yoga breaks. Observing the breath, bodily sensations, and the activity of the mind in posture—each of these practices enhances a student's ability to tune in to first his own and ultimately others' feelings.

Pause Breathing is a simple tool for increasing inner awareness. Begin by taking two slow deep breaths. Rather than another full inhalation, divide the next breath into three parts. Take about one third of an inhalation and pause; inhale another third and pause; complete the inhalation. Then exhale fully. Take a resting breath in between, and repeat the sequence. Do you notice any changes in the duration of the inhalation or exhalation? How do you feel when you finish that exercise?

Be sure to remind students that there is no right answer to these questions. It's a personal experience of what is going on inside them. (See Units 4 and 5 for lessons on attention and tuning in.)

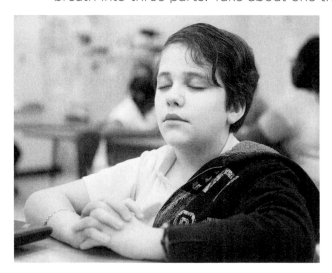

15-7   Pause Breathing

Face to Face: Social Engagement

Another aspect of social engagement involves responding to subtle cues from others. Consider a student who is barreling through the hallway, rushing to class. He is preoccupied with his mission, not paying attention to where he is going. Suddenly, he feels a jolt and is pushed into the lockers. Reflexively, he raises his fist, ready to take a swing at the offending body. Just before the blow reaches the large mass in his path, he looks up and sees the smiling face of a good friend. He reroutes the intended blow from the face to his friend's back-pack, giving him a sturdy shove without harm.

Why is it so much easier to forgive a friend than a stranger—even if they commit the same offense? It's because we have a history with a friend; we anticipate and perceive their actions as harmless. Because of something that neuroscientist Stephen Porges calls the social engagement system, our nervous system has the capacity to diffuse the sensation of threat and deactivate the signal for fight or flight.

This built-in form of radar helps us sift through the incoming data that can so easily be distorted. According to Porges (2005), the social engagement system is an autonomic response of the vagus nerve, which controls facial expression, language, tone, pitch, and rhythm of the voice. Using these tools, most individuals are able to discern the magnitude of a threat before responding (Porges, 2011). The capacity to distinguish a shriek of terror from a peal of laughter, or a friendly tease from an aggressive challenge, are all part of the social engagement system. By discerning intention via sensations from the vagus nerve, we are able to avoid full-blown fight-or-flight arousal. Similarly, by carefully controlling our volume, gestures, and tone of voice, many an argument can be averted. The social engagement system inhibits the limbic system from sounding the internal alarms (Porges, 2011).

Porges notes that face-to-face interaction is key in assessing another person's intentions and revealing our own. "Thus, familiar voices, calming gestures, and appropriate facial expressions can rapidly diffuse a possible physical conflict. . . . [A] well-defined social engagement system promotes social interactions . . . and promotes a sense of safety between people" (Porges, 2011, pp. 276–278).

Our capacity to perceive others' intention is stymied by many of the forms of

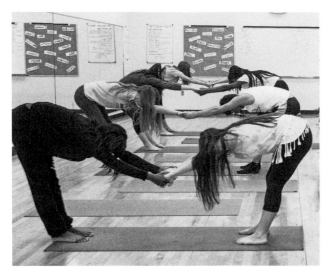

15-8   Partner Down Dog

communication that are common today. It's difficult to perceive how someone is feeling via texts, Facebook posts, or Twitter feeds. Misunderstandings that occur in online communications, for example, are much more difficult to correct because we can't hear the tone of voice or see the expression on the face of the sender. The less human our language becomes, the more difficult it is to access this information. Unfortunately, our youth rely increasingly on faceless, voiceless forms of communication.

Yoga breaks afford many opportunities to interact face to face. Partner poses require a great deal of social interaction and communication. Sharing someone's space without menace, helping to support a partner, offering encouragement, and confirming intention through words and gestures are all tools related to the social engagement system. Teaching children to interact in supportive and gentle ways is something that occurs in a natural environment when partnering in yoga.

Partnering and Social and Emotional Learning

When I was in sixth grade, my New England elementary school required coeducational square dancing. I wish I could tell you that I enjoyed it. Looking back, I see the rich opportunities this program offered for supporting social and emotional learning. We learned a great deal about self-awareness, self-management, social awareness, relationship skills, and responsible decision making:

- Boundaries—how to approach your partner (self-awareness, social awareness)
- Touch—how forcefully or gently to hold your partner's hands (self-management, social awareness)

- Teamwork—working together meant a successful dance; disregarding your partner resulted in feet being stomped on and instability (relationship skills, responsible decision making)
- Choice—if you had a partner who stood too close or was inattentive, you could choose a new partner for the next dance (self-management, responsible decision making)
- Consequences—if your behavior was deemed inappropriate by your partner, he or she would not accept another invitation to dance (relationship skills, responsible decision making)

Similarly, yoga breaks are an excellent tool to support social and emotional learning. Discovering relationships often involves experimentation with touch. In yoga breaks, we have the opportunity to teach adolescents ways to be physical with others without exceeding boundaries. We can encourage communication and respect while partnering.

If you stand too close to your partner in Tree Pose, you will destabilize one

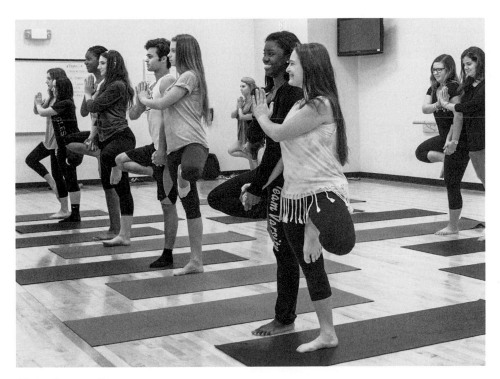

15-9   Partner Tree

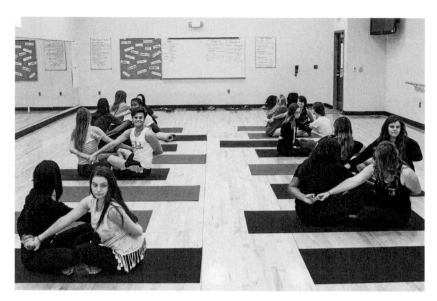

15-10   Partner Twist

another; too far and there's not enough support. This pose enhances self-management and social awareness.

Students quickly learn that if they pull their partner too far in seated Partner Twist, the pose will end abruptly and that person will be reluctant to partner with them next time. Being responsive to their partners, on the other hand, makes this posture a pleasant stretch for both participants. This is a lesson in relationship skills.

A posture like Flying Bats requires a great deal of concentration, communication, and negotiation. It teaches teamwork and patience. There is a personal

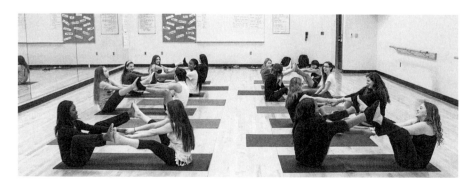

15-11   Flying Bats

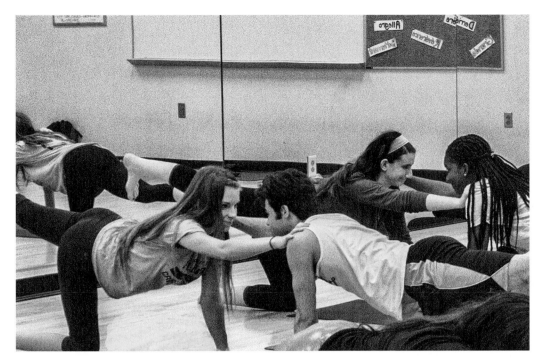

15-12   Partner Balance Beam

connection in this face-to-face posture that enhances social awareness and self-management skills.

Partner Balance Beam affords an opportunity to practice many of these social and emotional elements. This pose is a bilateral balance, which requires inward focus and calm (self-awareness). There are joint decisions to be made (responsible decision making) in terms of the positioning of partners and who supports whom first (relationship skills). Each partner must be aware of the other throughout the pose.

Yoga breaks help children feel more connected to themselves and to their community. Engaging students through acceptance and laughter makes classrooms friendlier and more conducive to learning. As children become more aware of their own inner feelings, they develop a greater capacity for empathy and compassion. Partner postures provide opportunities to interact face to face, learn to read others' intentions, and hone subtle cues that mitigate stress and enhance social interactions.

CHAPTER 16

Provide Tools for Success

IN THE PREVIOUS chapters, we've discussed the importance of feeling safe and establishing a sense of connection to oneself and others. Now we'll motivate students to practice yoga by demonstrating its benefits.

Most students want to succeed, but they may not know how. School performance has been linked to executive function; yoga breaks provide tools to improve students' ability to focus and stay on task. Young people may also be inspired by celebrities whose yoga practice has contributed to their own success. The supportive, positive communication strategies used in teaching yoga elevates students' self-esteem. By establishing consistent patterns for yoga breaks in your classroom, you mitigate anxiety and give students something to look forward to. Postures are also useful for easing transitions from one activity to another throughout the school day.

Yoga Breaks for Focus and Attention

Have you considered how many times in a day adults tell children to pay attention? Unfortunately, repeatedly asking distracted students to keep their minds on their work doesn't make their task any easier. Rather, it may contribute to increased frustration and poor self-esteem. If they knew how to pay attention, they would likely be doing so.

Few school curricula offer instruction on the process of paying attention. One of the definitions of yoga is "preventing [thought] from going around in circles" (White, 1996, p. 273), making it well suited to fill this gap. Balance poses, for example, are excellent tools for teaching focus and concentration. Supporting the weight of the body on one foot is nearly impossible while the mind is wandering.

You might try it right now: Stand on both feet. Begin reading a text, looking around the room, or mentally writing your to-do list. Elevate one foot an inch off the ground with all this mental activity. It's very difficult.

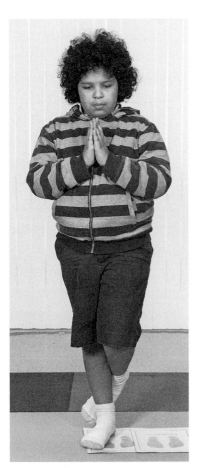

Now, let's make that exercise into a 1-minute yoga break: Tree Balance. Standing with the weight equally on both feet, gaze at a spot on the floor about five or six feet away—approximately your height in front of you. Take three slow, deep breaths, keeping your eyes fixed on this point. Slowly, shift your weight to the left foot. Keep your gaze and breathing steady while you touch your right toes behind your left heel. Once you feel steady, tuck the foot behind the ankle. If you lose your balance, lightly touch the toes down and hold there; lift the foot again only when you are ready. Release after 10 seconds. Stand again on both feet, without shifting your gaze. Slowly repeat on the other side for 10 seconds. When you are done, stand for a moment, still gazing at your spot, and take another deep breath.

Did you notice how much easier it was to balance with your eyes and mind focused on one spot? Even if balance was difficult, you probably felt the difference in your breathing. This pose is a striking way to teach children the power of the focused mind. Most students improve at balancing postures with regular practice, so it's self-rewarding.

16-1   Tree Balance

You will find introductory exercises for improving balance in Unit 3, and many others throughout the BREATHE FIRST curriculum.

Motivation Through Role Models

Most adolescents are highly motivated by something. Young people often expend a lot of energy in order to look or sound a certain way. Some invest their time in sports, drama, art, or music. Others spend hours working on school government, clubs, or community projects. Many are highly susceptible to following trends set by successful athletes, musicians, actors, or powerful political figures. Finding role models whose choices are responsible and healthy can be highly motivating.

Sometimes it helps to know that something that kids do in school is also cool. In Chapter 5 we discussed the increasing use of yoga among professional basketball and football players. The *Huffington Post* carries a lengthy online list of celebrities who love yoga, including Jennifer Aniston, Lady Gaga, Christy Turlington, Sting, Jessica Biel, Russell Brand, Gwyneth Paltrow, and Katy Perry ("Celebrities Who Swear by Yoga," 2014).

Musician and star of the television show *The Voice*, Adam Levine credits yoga for keeping his mind sharp and his body finely honed. In an interview for *Celebrity Workout*, Levine explained the demands of performing: "Playing a show before thousands of people is a highly unnatural state, . . . [but] when I get on the mat to do . . . yoga before the show, I come out physically relaxed" (Hooper, 2011).

Ohio congressman Tim Ryan (2012) practices and advocates for mindfulness training for schoolchildren. Hillary Rodham Clinton credits yoga and swimming for her abundant energy and good health (Heil, 2014). Michelle Obama also added yoga to her exercise regimen as she approached her 50th birthday (Alter, 2014).

In 2009, President and Mrs. Obama introduced yoga to the traditional Easter egg hunt and celebration, part of the first lady's Let's Move! initiative. Since then, over 30,000 children and adults from around the country have practiced yoga on the White House lawn each year in the Yoga Garden (Cullis, 2015).

Knowing that yoga is embraced by well-known individuals whose successes span multiple disciplines can be motivating to even the most reluctant exercisers.

Communication for Success

When examining ways to motivate students for school success, it's important to consider the choice of language that we use. Encouragement and praise can be transformative to students, especially those who experience little during a typical day.

At the 2015 Kripalu Yoga in Schools Symposium, Dr. Cynthia Zurchin explained the power of praise. She faced an uphill battle while serving as principal in a Pittsburgh elementary school. Fighting and abusive language were the norm; over half the student population had been suspended. It was an exhausting place to work and an impossible environment for learning.

Inspired by the book *Whale Done!* (Blanchard et al., 2002), Durbin began implementing a program of praise and encouragement. She coached faculty to ignore what students were doing wrong and focus instead on what they were doing right. Her goals were to "build trust, accentuate the positive, and when mistakes occur, redirect the energy." Over a 3-year period, she and her teachers learned to address the most challenging behavior issues with positive redirection.

In concert with these changes, Dr. Zurchin implemented the Yoga in Schools program, led by founder Joanne Spence, to promote calm and increase focus. Despite initial resistance, parents, teachers, and students learned to breathe and move mindfully, enhancing self-regulation skills and overall well-being. The school became a friendlier, kinder place—a healthier environment for learning.

These combined improvements resulted in measurable academic changes, with third grade proficiency increasing by 46% in reading and 60% in math. There were fewer incidents of tardiness and overall classroom attention improved. Most significant was the decrease in suspensions—from over 100 in 2006–2007 to 85 the next year, to 10 in 2008–2009 (Zurchin, 2015).

Consistency: Creating a Ritual

When children know what's coming, they can adapt more easily to it. Anticipating a pleasant break when their work is finished, for example, often motivates students to stay on task.

Setting up a schedule and following a consistent pattern for yoga breaks is especially helpful for anxious or highly stressed youth. By beginning and ending each class with a 1-minute break, or starting each class with a 5-minute calming lesson, you set a pattern that students can anticipate.

The same applies to the lessons themselves. Your students may find it helpful if you establish a ritual, a predictable routine, for the yoga break. Familiarity is reassuring.

You may substitute variations for each portion of your own routine, but here's a sample 5-minute routine:

1. Prepare the room and yourself: Ask everyone in the room to surrender or silence their phones. Dim the lights, play soft music, and take a deep breath to lower the pitch of your voice.

2. Huh Breath: Huh Breath signals the beginning of the lesson. Inhale and elevate the shoulders; exhale with a "huh" and drop the shoulders. Do this one to three times.

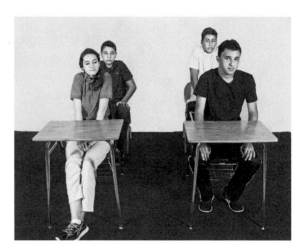

16-2   Huh Breath

3. Breathing: Start with soft belly breathing. Place one hand on your abdomen. Inhale and notice the movement—if any—in your belly. Do you notice movement anywhere else in your body when you breathe in? Exhaling, do the same. Take one to three soft breaths.

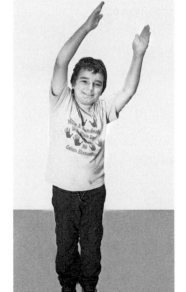

16-3   Half Moon Double Arm

4. Movement. This can be done seated and/or standing. Depending upon time available, include a variety of movements or just one moving pose.

Half Moon standing: Students stand next to their chairs with both arms overhead. They sway their arms from side to side freely. They lean to the right and hold, then to the left and hold. Do this one to three times. (This may be done seated at the desk.)

Folded Leaf: Turning sideways in their chairs, students place both hands on their thighs. They slowly slide down until their hands are dangling near their toes, and the head is resting on the knees. Inhale and exhale in the pose. Slowly slide the hands back up.

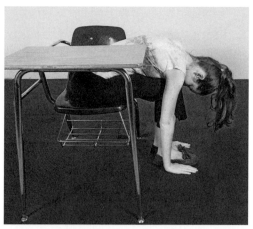
16-4   Folded Leaf

4. Mindful Attention. This is an opportunity to watch the mind. Here's an example: Balloon Thoughts: As you sit quietly, notice if a judgment or negative thought intrudes on your quiet. In your imagination, place that thought inside a big bright balloon. When you are ready, release the balloon, and watch that thought sail up toward the sky. Do this for 1 minute or less to start.

5. Relaxation: Your Special Place. Take a moment to imagine that you are in the most beautiful place in the world—in the mountains or by the sea, or a spot that no one has ever been before, somewhere peaceful and safe, where you feel secure and happy. This is your special place, where only you can go. Take three slow, soft belly breaths while you rest in your special place. When you are ready, open your eyes.

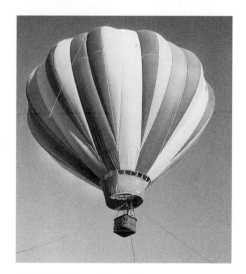
16-5   Balloon Thoughts

6. Huh Breath signals the conclusion of the lesson. Inhale and elevate the shoulders; exhale with a "huh" and drop the shoulders. Do this one to three times.

Once students are familiar with soft belly breathing, introduce other breathing exercises, one at a time. If you encounter students who need more movement, substitute standing or partner postures for the stillness portion. Follow with one quiet seated pose. You can still begin and conclude with Huh Breath.

You may discover that this is too much time away from classwork. If so, choose any one of those steps to do with your class, but do it regularly. Inform your students of your schedule, so they know that a break is in their near future.

Finding a system that works for your class is essential. And you are the person best equipped to make that determination. Once you have a ritual that you and your students are comfortable with, you can add or change portions of the routine as you choose (see Part V, the BREATHE FIRST curriculum).

Unwasting Time: Yoga for Transitions

It may be difficult for many educators to justify extensive breaks from academic work in each class. However, most teachers can identify periods of nonproductive time within their day.

Transitional periods are very difficult for lots of young people. Lunch periods, assemblies, and any unexpected schedule changes can be disturbing. Instead of moving directly from activity to activity, try using a few minutes to help your students settle down and refresh themselves. Taking a short yoga break to transition into class assignments may result in a far more productive period.

Time management, an element of executive function, is a skill that can be improved with practice. Most kids are masters at wasting time, at least when it comes to avoiding tasks that they don't enjoy. You can use yoga breaks to offer students additional tools for making the best use of their time.

For example, some of your students may arrive at school listless and unfocused after a long bus ride. When students come directly from lunch, they are often loud or distracted. Some teachers find those last few minute of the class, when their lesson is complete, empty time. You'll often have students who start off strong when class begins, but whose attention begins to fade halfway through.

These are ideal times for a short yoga break. Here are some examples from Unit 10 to help students transition back to work:

- Listless, unfocused: Follow Your Thumb. By watching their thumb with their eyes as they move their outstretched arm slowly from side to side, students redirect their focus.

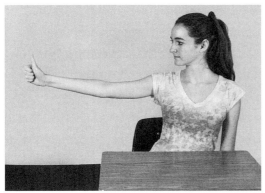

16-6   Follow Your Thumb

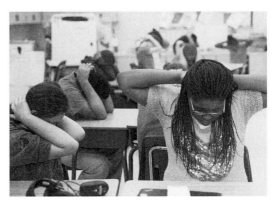

16-7   Bellows Breath 2 Chin Tuck

- After lunch: Bellows Breath 2 Chin Tuck. Clasping their hands behind their heads, students exhale and lower the chin toward the chest. Breathing gently while remaining in this position has a quieting effect on the nervous system, counteracting the noisy cafeteria.

- After an exam: Tense and Relax. Students begin by tightly squeezing their fists, shoulders, and facial muscles. With a deep exhalation, they relax all the muscles. Next they stretch their mouth and eyes, arms and fingers open wide, and then release.

- Wake-up break for mid-class: Palm Stretch and Lean. Interlacing the fingers, stretch the elbows straight, palms out. This feels good after writing or typing for a long time. Students stretch their arms overhead with an inhalation and lean to one side with an exhalation. They inhale to the center and repeat on the other side.

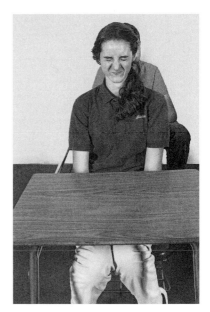

16-8   Tense and Relax

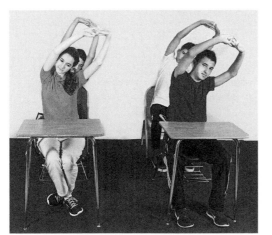

16-9   Palm Stretch and Lean

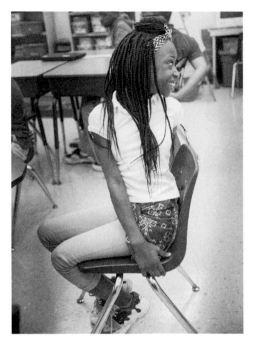

16-10 Seated Twist

• Empty time, end of class: Seated Pretzel. Before getting up from their seats at the end of class, students take a breath. Then they twist and pause in each direction.

Yoga breaks enhance students' ability to focus and stay on task. When celebrities and successful athletes tout the healthy benefits of yoga, many young people are motivated to try it themselves. The simplicity of the lessons and positive communication style increase students' experience of success. Providing a consistent routine and tools for easing transitions, yoga breaks support students throughout their school day.

CHAPTER 17

Foster Independence

I N THE PRECEDING chapters, we've explored a number of ways to empower young people through classroom yoga: creating a peaceful, safe space, engaging them in their community and the learning process, and providing tools to enhance their learning and social skills. By inviting students to stretch their bodies and minds, to use the information their bodies offer, and to exercise self-control, we foster independence.

Honing the ability to focus and redirect the mind is the path to freedom from distractions. I often remind my students that the world will not quiet or slow down because they want it to. It is their task to find a peaceful place within themselves, independent of the happenings around them. By learning to choose their response, even to events over which they have no control, they find an avenue to liberation.

The Courage to Fail

Learning and growing require taking an intellectual leap with unpredictable outcomes. Making mistakes, however, is not encouraged in our school culture.

The emphasis on test scores, GPA, and class rank supersedes curiosity and challenge in many scholastic settings. This fact has led to numerous episodes of cheating among students and even school personnel. It also discourages intellectual adventure; young people are loath to take courses or experiment with activities in which they aren't certain of success.

Yoga is a path of acceptance, encouraging all participants to value and to trust in their individual merit. In yoga breaks, we provide a safe space where children can fail without harm. When a child tries a difficult posture, even if she is unsuccessful, she learns to get up and try again. Each attempt teaches her something new about her body and her mind. If a child is fearful or physically less able, she can practice postures seated on the ground or in a chair. Gradually, under the guidance of a supportive teacher, she too can gain tools to address greater challenges.

By teaching children that it's okay to do something in a different way, as long as it's their own way, we lead them to greater self-awareness. By encouraging them to make and learn from their mistakes, we teach them that success is a process requiring commitment and effort. Yoga offers a new definition of fearlessness: a personal path leading to independence and resilience.

Independence Through Body Awareness

Most of our conscious brain is dedicated to focusing on the outside world: getting along with others and making plans for the future. However, that does not help us manage ourselves. Neuroscience research shows that the only way we can change the way we feel is by becoming aware of our *inner* experience and learning to befriend what is going on inside ourselves. (van der Kolk, 2014, p. 206)

In our society, there's a great deal of pressure to exceed the natural limits of our own bodies. Advertisements feature happy people taking medications so they can eat foods that upset their digestive system or go to work when their body is begging for a day of rest. Television series with contrived survival challenges glorify self-deprivation. Young people are often encouraged to "tough it out" rather than listen to and learn from the body. The motto "grin and bear it" encourages numbing themselves to their pain.

Pain is an indicator that something is wrong. Disregarding pain forces the body to intensify the message until it can no longer be ignored. When we adapt to extended periods of discomfort, we become desensitized to bodily warnings. This pattern, the general adaptation syndrome, can result in exhaustion, illness, or worse (Selye, 1974). Practicing movement with awareness teaches young people the importance of pain as a teacher (see Unit 12).

Sometimes children become numb to physical discomfort. PE teacher Donna Davis sees a lot of students who are driven to succeed at all costs. She incorporates yoga and stress management into her school dance program. A longtime dancer, Donna reflects:

> Dancing is hard on the joints. Cheerleaders and serious dancers come in with all these injuries. And there's a lot of emphasis on looking a certain way. That's not what this is about—I have kids of all shapes and sizes. Yoga is not about doing more pirouettes than the next girl; it's about inner awareness, self-esteem, doing it for yourself. I love the fact that it's not competitive, not about pushing past your edge. It's about finding your own comfort. (personal communication, October 17, 2014)

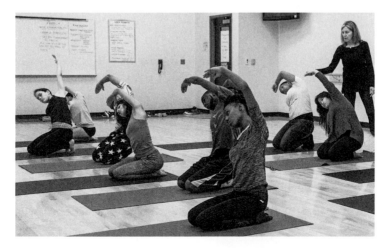

17-1   Finding Comfort

Rather than "no pain, no gain," a better motto in yoga breaks is "no pain, no pain." Starting with the body, students learn to tune into sensations and identify their feelings. As they become more adept at feeling their bodily sensations, they begin to notice ways that their feelings are affected—by what they do and say; by what others do and say to them; and by how they think about themselves and others.

Learning to recognize the subtle messages that make them feel a certain way, students develop a sense of control over their responses to the world around them. They recognize where their feelings come from and what they can do to change them (see Appendix 3).

Rosana Giani, the parent of a very bright and tenderhearted fifth grader, shared her observations about her daughter's response to feelings:

> When Angelina was introduced to yoga with you several years ago, she was having trouble adjusting to a new teacher. Her teacher was very loud and very critical; it was an unpleasant classroom experience. She didn't want to go to school.
>
>   Some people are able to disregard "mean" behaviors but others need to learn how to do that. My daughter is highly sensitive and she absorbs other people's feelings—good or bad. After learning in yoga how to relax and turn inward, she was able to tune out the loud teacher and the negativity she projected in the classroom. (personal communication, August 8, 2015)

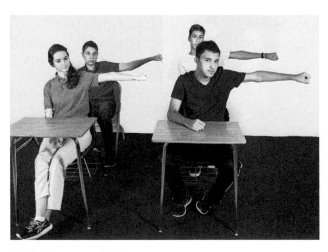

17-2   Tense and Relax

Tense and Relax is a useful exercise for releasing unnecessary holding. And it can be done without making a sound. Like progressive muscle relaxation or body scanning, it's a system for perusing the body, noticing how it feels inside, and consciously releasing tension. It's easiest to start with the extremities—straightening the arm and making a tight fist, and then letting it go; squeezing the toes, and then relaxing them. The shoulders are another good place to work: Shrug them up to the ears, and then drop; draw the shoulder blades together in back, and release. Squeeze the eyes and facial muscles together, tense the fists, and relax. With practice, specific muscles throughout the body can be isolated—calves, thighs, upper arms, and so on.

This sequence helps teach students a great deal about restrictions within their bodies. It's also useful for letting go tension that gets absorbed from unpleasant circumstances (see Unit 2).

Independence in Social Intercourse: Touch and Boundaries

As students become better observers of their own bodies, they can apply this knowledge in social settings.

There are inherent benefits that comes from appropriate physical contact with others. Most people find comfort in touch. Independent of one's language abilities, a gentle touch calms, a pat on the back encourages, an embrace soothes, a hi five welcomes. Not surprisingly, research using fMRI revealed that a touch on the arm from a friend during a stressful episode reduced the response of the amygdala, the brain's internal alarm system (Coan, Schaefer, & Davidson, 2006).

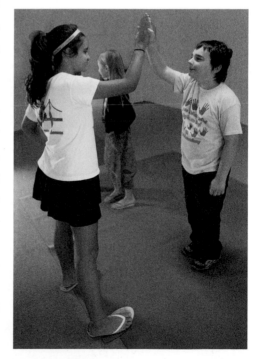

Many adolescents are confused about touch. Whether they are curious, fearful, overzealous, or naive, it's a complex topic. Experimentation is likely during this period. Boundaries are tested. Yoga breaks are useful for teaching young people that touch is healing and can be an expression of kindness. It's also important that students learn to say no to unwanted touch, firmly and with authority. Yoga postures teach students to stand up for themselves in varying circumstances (see Unit 12).

Partner strength postures teach students about touch in another way: They are stronger with a partner, but also more vulnerable. A good example is partner Side Angle pose (see Unit 12). Standing back

17-3   Hi Five

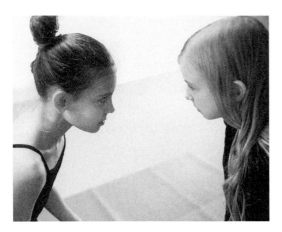

17-4   Boundaries

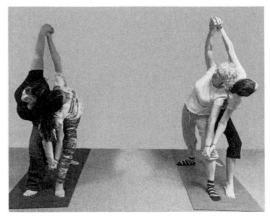

17-5   Partner Side Angle Pose

to back, moving in tandem, they form a supportive wall for one another. As long as each respects the other's comfort and limitations, their partnership is grounding. They also must learn to part with grace.

Even those who may not easily sense how others feel can learn to make better social choices in terms of physical boundaries through their own body pre-

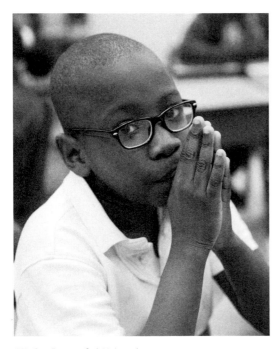

17-6   Peaceful Friend

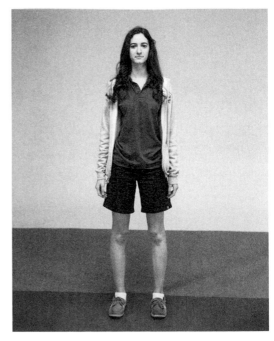

17-7   Mountain Stance

sentation. By practicing specific poses, students can be coached about the impact that their body positions have on others. To present oneself as a peaceful friend, for example, use quiet Tree Hands. When feeling threatened, assume Mountain Stance. If during an agitated encounter their hands seem to take on a life of their own, they can interlace their fingers and stretch the palms down; then relax their hands by their side (see Sense of Self Lessons, 5, How Do You Present Yourself in Unit 11).

Independence Through Self-Awareness: Mind the Gap

In her book for children with high-functioning autism, Catherine Faherty describes a strategy called Mind the Gap. After traveling on the London subway system and hearing the term "mind the gap" called out at each station, Jack Wall of the Charlotte TEACCH Center was inspired by this concept. He describes the gap as that moment between a stressful incident and the response it provokes (Faherty, 2000, p. 262).

Many individuals with ASD are plagued with unpredictable behaviors. Meltdowns sometimes come on so quickly that the child having the incident is as surprised as those around him. This contributes to the frustration of being out of control. Faherty explains that these young people often miss the warning signs that others use to avoid going over the emotional edge. The gap, she explains, is "the time a choice can be made as to what actions to take" (Faherty, 2000, p. 262). She suggests using visual cues or social stories to help students explore the signals of stress that precede their outbursts. Then work with them to develop alternative responses to these signals, thus averting unwanted behaviors.

Although Mind the Gap is a behavior technique designed for children and teens with high-functioning autism, it is useful for teaching many young people who struggle with self-regulation. The first step is learning to recognize the sensations that precede a loss of control. These may include shallow breathing, tightness in the jaw, or a burning sensation at the back of the neck. Although different for each person, students can learn to identify warning signals that often precede an explosive reaction.

Developing alternative strategies is the next step. Instead of reflexively hitting, pushing, or storming off, they have a choice. There is a moment, a pause between trigger and response. What might they do instead?

For example, a student may begin to notice that his hands get sweaty or he has a funny feeling in his stomach before emotional outbursts. With practice, he may find that sitting down and taking three cooling breaths (see Unit 12) changes how he feels. The sweating or the funny feelings begin to subside, and he's able to redirect his behavior. Now he has a personal tool (see Appendix 3).

Ali Smith, executive director of the Holistic Life Foundation, provides direct yoga instruction to youth in underserved communities. He finds that yoga helps middle schoolers curb aggressive behaviors. "They learn to take a breath, instead of flying off the handle or belittling others. By pausing first, they react with more awareness. They take their yoga practice from the mat to their desks" (personal communication, October 15, 2014).

An exercise that has helped many of my students to regain control is Fast Twister, and it takes just a minute. Students stand and sway from side to side. Quickly they pick up speed, letting their arms fly out to the sides. Then they slow it down. Again fast! And slow it down.

Respiration accelerates with the fast twist, and slows as the motion slows. These respiratory shifts and the cross-patterning movements of the arms help regulate the nervous system (Hannaford, 2005).

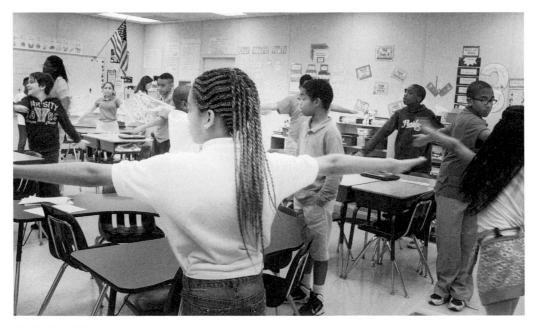

17-8   Fast Twister

Practicing these techniques during a quiet time in the day makes them more easily summoned when needed. By learning to recognize the difference between tension and relaxation within their own bodies, students learn to recognize the warning signals that precede meltdowns or unwanted behaviors. In this way, they can change their responses and regulate their own behaviors.

Outlets for Frustration

Frustration isn't always obvious, and it looks different from person to person. Sometimes it's clear that a child is nearing the edge of his tolerance: His face turns red, his jaws are clenched, and his respiration is fast and shallow. Some children, however, don't reveal anything until they explode in a fit of anger, tears, or aggression.

Providing students with outlets for movement, laughter, and making noise will often reduce their levels of anxiety and irritability. Releasing tension at regular intervals throughout the day may prevent escalation of these feelings. Students who practiced yoga in combination with social-emotional skills during their school days had lower levels of anger and were less likely to harbor vengeful thoughts than their peers (Frank et al., 2014). Yoga and mindfulness programs have shown reduced anger (Khalsa et al., 2012) and less anxiety (Mendelson et al., 2010) among school participants.

A simple yoga break to release frustration is Shake Shake Shake. This exercise, performed seated or standing, moves one side of the body at a time. Students begin by shaking out the fingers of one hand, then the whole hand and wrist. Next they shake the arm, followed by the shoulder. This sequence is then repeated on the other side. Starting again on one side, they shake their toes, foot, ankle, knee, thigh, and hip. This is repeated on the other leg. Finally, students shake their hair and, if balance is not an issue, their heads. If time is limited, they may shake both sides of the body simultaneously.

By the time all of the shaking is going on, most students are giggling or laughing. There's an increase in respiration and heart rate from the movement. This mini-workout is a great tool for preventing the buildup of frustration (see Unit 8).

A brief version of Shake Shake Shake is called Shake It Out, which combines all the shaking at one time, standing or seated. Other quick tension relievers

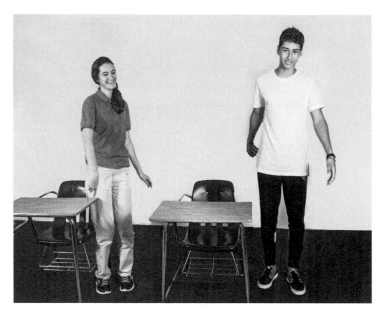

17-9   Shake It Out

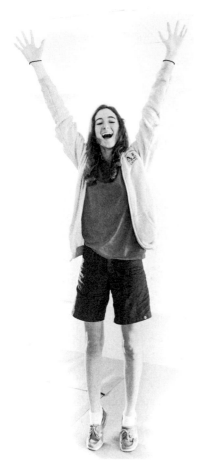

17-10   Volcano

include Volcano (see Unit 8), which starts in a squat and ends with a leap, and Rag Doll (see Unit 10), a standing forward fold. You'll find lots more postures for releasing tension throughout the BREATHE FIRST curriculum.

Another exercise that I've practiced with children of all ages is the High Striker. It's based on a carnival attraction, which uses a mallet to strike a puck at the bottom of a tower. With sufficient force, the puck travels up to ring a bell near the top of the tower.

You can combine this exercise with a discussion about ways to release tension or frustration. How do students release these feelings? Do they find themselves on occasion exploding inappropriately because they've let things build up inside? High Striker is an opportunity to release a lot of emotional junk.

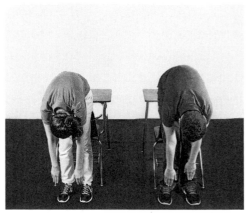

17-11   Rag Doll

To begin, ask students to survey their body for tension. Standing next to their desks, ask them to place their hands on their neck, shoulders, or lower back—somewhere that they feel tight. Then gather that tension in their hands and throw it down on the ground. This can be repeated up to three times, either returning to the same place or finding tension in another area of the body. This is all done without a sound.

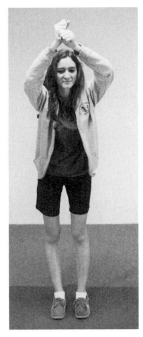

Now, direct the students to gather up all the tension that they've thrown onto the ground into a heap. They can do that with their hands or by moving it around with their feet. They pick up their imaginary striker, something that looks like a croquet mallet, and take a deep breath in. Then, exhaling with a loud "huh" sound, they slam that striker toward the ground, sending their tension flying up into the air. Repeat up to three times. To be sure that all of the tension has been released, students may stomp on the pile and scatter away the last bits of tension. To conclude, they stand quietly for a moment and observe their bodies.

17-12   High Striker

This entire sequence can be repeated, focusing on releasing anger or other emotions (see Unit 7). Yoga breaks provide opportunities for students to hone their own communication skills. In addition to creating an environment for nonjudgmental listening, Unit 7 provides lessons for releasing frustration and negative feelings.

Controlling Volume: Noisy Versus Quiet

Many teachers find that if they give their students a small amount of freedom, they abuse it. When students work in small groups, for example, the noise level can elevate quickly. To prevent this potential explosion of sound, many teachers avoid these situations by confining students to seat work. The problem with this model is that learning is actually enhanced by social interaction and movement. In addition, students miss a valuable opportunity to monitor their own behavior.

Yoga breaks can aid students in learning to modulate their volume (Goldberg, 2013). Start with an agreed-upon signal for quiet and one for noisy. I usu-

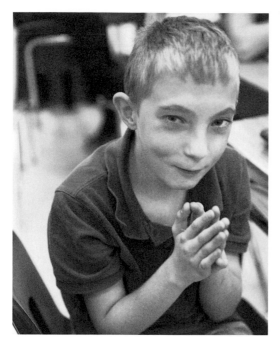

17-13   Quiet Hands

ally use my hands. Begin with your palms together, and ask the group to practice silence. Once that is mastered, choose a syllable such as "oh" or "ahh" to begin. As you widen your hands, students may escalate their volume. As you bring them closer together, they grow gradually quieter. When the hands come together, silence is restored. Begin the practice with brief periods of noise, followed by brief silences.

Most students relish the opportunity to be noisy. Explain that this exercise will be repeated only if students respect the hand signal for silence. Otherwise, quickly terminate the activity. Remember, to teach children to distinguish between these extremes, you have to let them get really loud. So be sure that you are prepared for lots of noise before beginning these practices.

After regular practice, allow students to take turns leading this activity, giving them an opportunity to teach and practice cooperation. You can use this signal during other class activities, as needed, to cue the class when they are getting too loud. Students are often scolded for being too loud. Some lack the skills to control their volume. Others may simply not realize how noisy their voices have become. Others may use noise to release frustration or anger. Teaching children to switch from noisy to quiet is not only fun, but also offers tools in self-awareness. Show your students that by exercising self-control, they earn greater freedom within the classroom.

Resetting the Boiling Point

One constant that I have observed as a teacher of all age groups is that frustration generally boils up over time. It may appear to come on suddenly, but there is more often a growing swell of anger or anxiety that ultimately erupts into a meltdown or aggressive outburst. As Sapolsky explains, "psychological stress . . . is exacerbated if there is no outlet for frustration, no sense of control, no social support and no impression that something better will follow. . . . A person will become less hypertensive when exposed to painfully loud noise if she believes she can . . . lower the volume; she has a sense of control" (2003, pp. 87–90).

Learning to use appropriate outlets for frustration gives young people a sense of control. This is inherent in feeling independent. Having the freedom to move around and release muscular tension, to take a few deep breaths and regulate their nervous systems, to have a short conversation or some quiet time to reassess their feelings—these tools can prevent the buildup of stress that may lead to aggression, depression, or withdrawal.

For individuals with extreme sensory irregularities or limited language skills, processing frustration is even more difficult. Here physical releases through gentle or vigorous movement are especially empowering.

I'm a tea drinker, and I've noticed that it doesn't always take the same amount of time to boil water. It depends on how much water is in the kettle, what temperature it was when I put the kettle on, and on which burner I place the kettle—all this variation just in making a cup of tea.

With children, there are many factors determining their level of "boil." It depends on conditions that are both internal and external: How long is their internal fuse? What or who is provoking them? How were they feeling just before the episode began?

Each of us has an internal boiling point—a moment when our body shifts into full-blown hypervigilance, fight-or-flight, or meltdown mode. This process is a response of the autonomic nervous system to the stimuli from within and outside our bodies. The physiological properties of the response are consistent in many ways—accelerated heart rate, fast shallow breathing, sweating palms, a sick feeling in the pit of the stomach. But the moment when we each reach that precipice may vary greatly. Have you noticed that your internal fuse is much shorter after a poor night's sleep? When you are preoccupied with work or family responsibilities? When you've had a fight with your spouse or mother? When you're hungry? Just like my teakettle, there are many factors that contribute to the speed of the boil—and its intensity.

Usually it takes my teakettle about 5 minutes to come to a full boil. Sometimes I put the kettle on and leave the room. My husband, seeing the kettle untended, shuts it off. I return and turn it on. He comes back and shuts it off.

If we turn it on and off, on and off, it's going to take much longer for the kettle to achieve a full head of steam. We can coach children to do the same with their frustration. Instead of letting things build and build until their fuses becomes so short that they blow, they can learn to shut off the source of tension, just like lowering the heat under the kettle. By interjecting periods of guided or self-calming through mindful breathing, movement, and focused attention, students can learn to reset their internal fuses to prevent or deter explosive bursts of rage, frustration, and anxiety. These tools can serve young people throughout their lives.

You will find additional tools for fostering independence in Appendixes 2 and 3.

PART V

BREATHE FIRST YOGA AND MINDFULNESS CURRICULUM
A Creative Relaxation Program for Social and Emotional Learning

BREATHE FIRST is a yoga and mindfulness curriculum for meeting your students where they are; reducing stress through breathing, movement, and stillness; improving learning readiness, attention, and focusing skills; and enhancing social and emotional learning (SEL) and increasing self-regulation skills. The goal is to make your classroom a calmer, happier, healthier place for you and your students.

You may follow the curriculum in its entirety or pick and

choose from among the over 200 practices and exercises offered in the twelve units. Many of the lessons combine a series of postures. Use the full lesson as a 5-minute "flow" or select individual exercises from the lessons for 1-minute yoga breaks.

CHAPTER 18

Guidelines for Teachers

How We Breathe

When we flip through magazines, watch television, or view Instagram, we are inundated with food, fashion, cars, and home furnishings. This type of consumption occupies a great deal of our time, money, and imagination. But are any of these needed to survive? Some people endure months or even years without adequate shelter or clothing. Mahatma Gandhi survived 21 days without eating. It's possible to live for a week without water. So, what is essential?

Breathing is vital. Most people can survive only a few minutes without permanent damage to the oxygen-deprived brain. It doesn't cost a thing to breathe. We don't even have to think about it—the body breathes for us. But there is an art and science to breathing in the most efficient manner.

The respiratory function is unusual in that it is part of both autonomic and voluntary systems. The rate of respiration affects the speed of the heartbeat, which alters the nervous system. As we become proficient at observing our breath—its speed, depth, volume, location—we become better able to regulate many aspects of body and mind.

Fast, shallow breathing usually indicates anxiety or stress, while slow, rhythmic breathing generally reflects a calmer state of mind and body. Stressful or joyful events, real or imagined, frequently change the rate and quality of respiration.

If you've ever watched a scary movie, you already know a lot about the relationship between breathing and emotions. As soon as the evil villain appears, your breathing and heart rate accelerate. You suck in your breath when he creeps behind his potential victim and hold it while he raises his weapon. Your breath explodes in a scream when he strikes. When the hero finally overcomes the villain, you heave a huge sigh of relief (Goldberg, 2013). It's only then that your breathing returns to normal and your heart stops its erratic pounding.

Clearly, your breathing changes in response to what's going on around you. The inverse is also true: How you breathe alters your nervous system, and that affects your physical and emotional state. "Abnormal breathing patterns can stimulate autonomic reactions associated with panic attacks," explains yoga anatomist David Coulter (2001, p. 90). In fact, "poor breathing habits . . . produce anxiety and chronic overstimulation of the sympathetic nervous system" (p. 90). Research by Philippot, Chapelle, and Blairy (2002) found that breathing patterns account for 40% of the changes in an individual's sensation of anger, fear, sadness and joy.

Fortunately, Coulter points out, changing the rate and quality of respiration—slowing down and deepening the breath—can also slow the heart rate, lower blood pressure, and stabilize the nervous system. And this is something that we can learn to do. "Our ability to control respiration consciously gives us access to autonomic functions that no other system of the body can boast" (Coulter, 2001, p. 90).

Yoga breathing has become an effective treatment for psychiatric disorders such as anxiety and PTSD (Cabral et al., 2011). According to Brown, Gerbarg, and Muskin, breathing at the rate of five to six breaths per minute, described as "coherent breathing, is a safe and easily accessible method to reduce anxiety, insomnia, depression, fatigue, anger, aggression, impulsivity, inattention, and symptoms of PTSD. . . . [It] has no adverse effects, and can be used in children" (2009, p. 81).

Coulter (2001) cautions against forcing respiration to an unnaturally slow pace, as that also may contribute to stress. Even doubling the length of the exhalation relative to the inhalation, which usually triggers parasympathetic dominance of the nervous system, will not derail a meltdown once an individual is in full-blown stress mode.

That's why it's important to practice rhythmic, steady breathing in a safe, comfortable setting. This gives students a tool for slowing the body down anywhere. The more frequently they practice, the more easily they can access the breath as a means for self-regulation during adversity.

How To Use This Curriculum

BREATHE FIRST Yoga and Mindfulness Curriculum adheres to the principles of Creative Relaxation: Create a peaceful space, engage the student, provide tools for success, and foster independence. Each unit is designed to expand on a theme, derived from the acronym BREATHE FIRST: B, breathing; R, relaxation; E, exercise; A, attention; T, tuning in and tuning out; H, heart opening; E, expressing; F, fun; I, intention; R, reset; S, sense of self; T, in touch. Aspects of the first four units, Breathing, Relaxation, Exercise, and Attention, are included in each subsequent unit.

The program is designed to be implemented during the school day in brief segments of 1 to 5 minutes in duration. Each of the 12 thematic units contains breathing lessons, movement, relaxation, and mindful awareness exercises, as well as practices for discussion or writing based upon the unit theme. You may use each lesson in the unit, or single exercises from within the lessons as individual yoga breaks. Unit 2, for example, contains calming sequences from both seated and standing positions. Each of these lessons contains 10 poses that may be practiced individually or as a series. There are over 200 postures and activities in this book—enough to practice a different one each day of the school year.

The practices and lessons within the units include discussion, research, social science, literature and poetry, physical science, and math, lending them to inclusion in mainstream class curricula as well as art, music, physical education, and SEL programs.

As you work with the curriculum, let your students' needs help guide your choices. For students who have difficulty with quiet sitting, select the movement portions of each unit. You can always come back to the mindfulness exercises at a later time. With less than a minute, select one breathing or one standing exercise. Should students be reluctant to get out of their seats, start with discussion or practices from the desk. With a class that really needs to move, choose from the varied postures in Unit 3, Exercise. You may find that some of the practices supplement your academic course material. SEL skills are interwoven within each unit.

Use each of the 12 units for as long as you choose before moving on to the next. Some teachers select one lesson each day, with a new unit each week or two. If you teach health or SEL classes, you may choose to combine many of the lessons within the unit for an extended classroom practice each week. Some teachers pick and choose from specific postures, lessons, or discussion topics within each unit to fit into their existing curricula.

If you have a group that is especially in need of relaxation skills, you may prefer to work with lessons from the Breathing and Relaxation units (1 and 2) for a month or more. Some students have difficulty with an unfamiliar routine, so you may choose a single lesson from one unit and repeat it daily for multiple weeks. Your students may need more social engagement, so group practices and partner poses may be most beneficial for them. Others may find the quiet meditative practices in each unit a welcome change from their noise-filled day.

Despite the emphasis on breathing exercises in this curriculum, you may choose to practice the movement elements exclusively. As discussed in Chapter 11, movement improves learning readiness and overall responsiveness among children (Hannaford, 2005). As explained by Stephen Porges, simply changing one's posture can trigger the calming mechanisms in the body (personal communication, June 5, 2015).

In addition, some students have difficulty connecting to their breath. Instruction in this area creates additional self-consciousness, confusion, or even stress. Fortunately, the postures alone will change the rhythm and tempo of your students' breathing. Energizing and strength poses will accelerate their respiration; calming and balance poses will slow it. Heart-opening postures will increase the depth of their inhalations; forward folds will lengthen their exhalations. By practicing the movement portion of yoga breaks, your students will expand their respiratory range and awareness.

For Teachers: Before You Begin

The following guidelines will help you integrate the principles of Creative Relaxation in every lesson.

CREATE A PEACEFUL SPACE

Peaceful Community

With the first lesson, introduce students to the Guidelines for Classroom Yoga Breaks (see Chapter 14). Discuss all 10 if you have time. Give special emphasis to number 1, "Be kind—Do no harm to others or yourself." This guideline underlies all postures and practices in yoga breaks. Periodically revisit the full list. You may select one of these guidelines for an in-depth discussion during each of the first 10 units.

To promote a peaceful environment, encourage quiet time during breathing postures and relaxation exercises.

Keep It Safe: Contraindications and Modifications

Moving yoga breaks are not suitable for students who have injuries or are unwell. If you are uncertain about a student's condition, he or she should practice postures from a seated position only or use only the nonmoving portions of the unit. Keeping one hand on the desk or chair is recommended until students become proficient at balancing exercises.

Inversions

Inversions are any position in which the head is below the level of the heart. Since yoga breaks are practiced seated or standing by the desk, the inversions most frequently used are Rag Doll and Folded Leaf, both forward bends. Avoid inversions if the student has a history of seizures, heart disease, spinal, back, or neck injury or instability, or headache, or after eating or drinking. Hypertension, high blood pressure, elevated intracranial pressure, stroke, glaucoma, detached retina, carotid artery stenosis, congestive heart failure, and hiatal hernia all contraindicate inversions (Cole, cited in Rosen, 2002).

These postures can be modified so that students do not lower the head

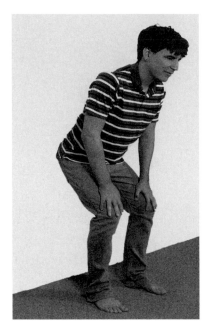 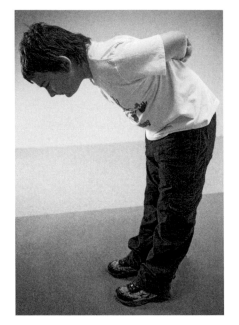

18-1 Half Rag Doll Bent Knees   18-2 Half Rag Doll

below heart level by supporting the head in the hands in seated folds. In standing forward bends, press the hands into the thighs, soften the knees, and extend the elbows to prevent lowering the head beyond chest level. Another option is to hold the elbows behind the back and hinge forward less than halfway.

Back Bending

Guide students to keep a long spine and not to drop their heads back in backward-bending, heart-opening postures. Ask them to imagine holding a softball at their throat notch to prevent compressing the spine at the back of the neck.

ENGAGE STUDENTS

Meet Them Where They Are

When beginning your program of classroom yoga breaks, keep it simple. Choose postures that are easy for your students. You may add more challenging or complex positions gradually, especially if it helps maintain students' interest.

Use brief lessons and conclude each task while students are experiencing success. This improves self-esteem and increases their willingness to try it again.

Adapt the Pace

Yoga breaks make it easier to meet your students where they are with the varied tempos of activities within each unit. When students walk into class boisterous or antsy, it may be difficult for them to sit still for meditation or focusing exercises. They would be better served by energizing postures or silly lessons.

If your class is lethargic, start with quiet seated breathing exercises or calming exercises. If you try to push them into more movement than they feel ready for, they will likely resist. Observe your students and select a starting place that is suitable for the moment. If you meet them where they are energetically, everyone's frustration will be lessened.

Use your voice—volume, tempo, pitch, projection—as well as your choice of postures to create a pace. To energize students, increase the volume and power behind your voice. Soften your voice and slow it down for calming postures.

TOOLS FOR SUCCESS

Keep It Positive

For many individuals, positive reinforcement is an effective tool for mitigating unproductive behaviors. The simple postures and breathing techniques included in the BREATHE FIRST curriculum afford every student an opportunity to shine at some point in their day. If a student has been talking, acknowledge him when he is quiet. Instead of lavishing attention on those who are not participating, praise students who are. By vigilantly rewarding only those behaviors that you wish to reinforce, you motivate students and redirect their behaviors in positive ways.

Transitions

Creating a schedule and using consistent starting and ending postures for each lesson creates a smoother transition into yoga breaks during class time. Let students know, for example, that class will begin and end with a 2-minute break.

For students who have difficulty changing from one activity to another, select one posture or breathing exercise to serve as a transitional cue. You may use this for the entire class or with individual students.

FOSTER INDEPENDENCE

Remind students that in yoga breaks, comfort is essential—no pain, no pain. There are many acceptable variations of each pose, and it is their task to do nothing that causes them harm. If a position does not feel suitable for their body, it is best to come out of the posture and focus on soft belly breathing.

Empower your students to make responsible choices by observing their feelings. This is the process of self-regulation.

The following units are organized around the 12 fundamental principles of BREATHE FIRST: breathing, relaxation, exercise, attention, tuning in and tuning out, heart opening, expressing, fun, intention, reset, sense of self, and in touch. Each unit includes a description of the principle, followed by practices and lessons in language that you can use with your students in the classroom.

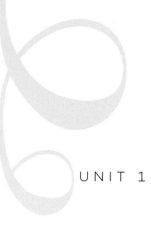

UNIT 1

Breathing

THE BREATH IS our constant companion throughout life. Our first independent act is to take a breath. When we expire, we release our final breath.

In the BREATHE FIRST curriculum, you will learn breathing techniques for self-regulation. By learning to breathe first, you pause, rebalance your nervous system, and begin to control the pace of your life. Instead of simply reacting to events, breathe first; then proceed with enhanced awareness.

The Anatomy of Breathing

Breathing is an exchange of gases; oxygen is inhaled and carbon dioxide is exhaled. The primary muscle of respiration is the diaphragm, which separates the chest and abdominal cavities. This thin sheet of muscle and tendon is attached to the sternum in front, the ribcage at the sides, and the spine in back. The diaphragm is generally active in inhalation and passive in exhalation. With the in-breath, its umbrella-shaped dome contracts and descends, increasing pressure within the abdominal cavity. This causes the abdominal wall to distend and the lower ribs to widen. When the diaphragm relaxes, it retracts up toward the rib cage, pushing air out of the lungs. This is exhalation. The abdomen and chest return to their normal shape.

Normally, breathing is in and out through the nose. The small hairs in the nostrils prevent particles of dust or debris from entering the lungs. During physical exertion or increased stress, the abdominal muscles become active during exhalation; respiration becomes faster and often more shallow; mouth breathing may result. This is a normal response when the nervous system is under sympathetic dominance, fight or flight. Breathing in this manner for extended periods, however, may deplete the body's energy reserves—compromising digestion, endocrine function, and the immune system.

Sometimes mouth breathing becomes habitual, especially during periods of great stress. Slowing the rate of respiration and nasal breathing generally have a calming effect on the nervous system.

Unless otherwise instructed, remind students to breathe in and out through the nostrils during yoga breaks. If a student cannot breathe through the nose, do not accentuate this issue; it's more important that he or she breathes comfortably in whatever way is accessible.

Practice 1: Visual Breathing

Create a rhythm for breathing using the Hoberman Sphere. Hold the sphere at the level of the abdomen. Illustrate the speed and depth of breathing by expanding the sphere with the inhalation and compressing it with the exhalation. Experiment with slight variations in the breathing patterns that you model.

Invite students to take turns leading the breathing lessons with the sphere.

Practice 2: The Diaphragm

The respiratory diaphragm looks something like a jellyfish. Its rounded "head" sits just below the lungs, and its tendrils reach down to attach on the ribs, sternum, and all the way down to the lumbar spine.

1. Draw an illustration of the diaphragm and adjacent organs during inhalation and exhalation.
2. What happens to the abdominal organs with an inhalation? With an exhalation?

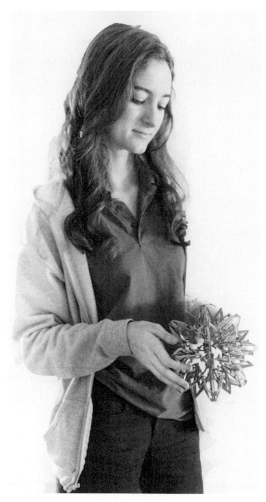

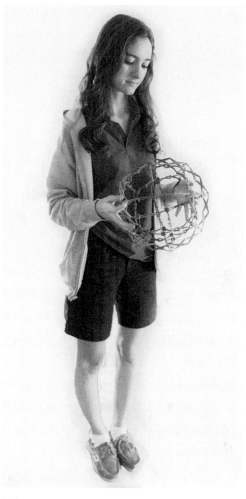

Hoberman Sphere Contracted

Sphere Expanded

3. How does this affect the shape of the abdominal area with inhalation and exhalation?

Practice 3: The Language of Respiration

Many terms in everyday language relate to the process of breathing. When you have a great idea, you're "inspired"; when you see something extraordinary, it "takes your breath away."

1. Can you think of other words or phrases related to respiration?

2. Write a haiku or sentence using one set of these antonyms: inhalation and exhalation; inspiration and expiration; inhale and exhale; inspire and expire.

3. Write a poem or paragraph using one of these metaphors (or others of your choice related to respiration): catch my breath, knocked the breath out of me, waiting breathlessly.

Breathing Lessons

1. Huh Breath three times: Use this breath to start and end each lesson (standing or seated). Works well as a transition between activities in class.

   a. Inhaling, shrug your shoulders up toward your ears.

   b. Exhaling, drop them down with a "huh."

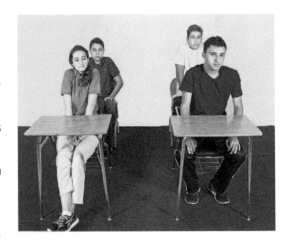

Huh Breath

2. Soft belly breathing: Relaxed breathing has an effortless quality. Have you ever watched a baby asleep in its crib? Its little tummy elevates with each breath in and lowers with each breath out. Try it now three times.

   a. Inhaling through the nose, fill your belly like a balloon.

   b. Exhaling through the nose, your belly slowly deflates.

   Lightly interlace your fingers and let the palms rest against your belly. Watch your fingers while you breathe three times.

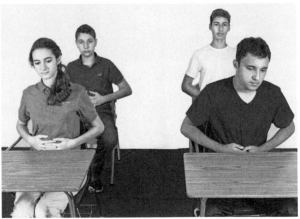

Soft Belly Breathing

   c. Notice if your fingers move apart when you inhale.

d. Do they come closer together when you exhale?

e. As your breathing deepens, do you experience more movement in your belly?

Remember not to force the belly in or out, because that increases tension. Instead, simply observe your breathing without trying to change it.

3. Rate of respiration: The way you breathe affects how you feel.

   • Soft belly breath

      a. Inhaling through the nose, fill your belly like a balloon.

      b. Exhaling through the nose, your belly slowly deflates.

      Make this a slow, easy breath. How does it feel? Repeat two more times.

   • Rapid breathing: Now consciously accelerate the rate of your breathing.

      c. Breathe in faster through your nose.

      d. Breathe out faster through your nose.

      Repeat five or six more times. Is it difficult to breathe in this way? How does it make you feel?

   • Mouth breathing: Now breathe rapidly through your mouth.

      e. Breathe in rapidly through your mouth.

      f. Breathe out rapidly through your mouth.

      Repeat three more times. How does it make you feel?

   • Soft belly breath: Once again, slow down your breathing.

      g. Inhaling through the nose, fill your belly like a balloon.

      h. Exhaling through the nose, your belly slowly deflates.

      Make this a slow, easy breath. In what ways is this different from the accelerated breath? Repeat until your respiration slows down. How do you feel?

4. Parachute breath (standing or seated): Start with your arms hanging at your sides. Inhale, turn the palms out, and sweep the arms up alongside you and overhead, palms touching. Exhaling, turn

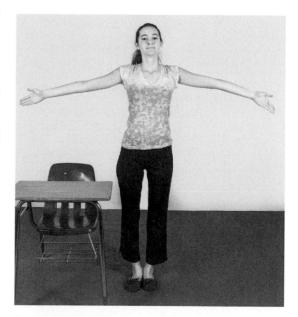

Parachute Breath

the palms out and float them back down to your sides. Repeat three to five times.

5. Elbow pumping (standing or seated): Rest your right palm on your right shoulder, left hand on your left shoulder. Inhale, open the elbows out to the sides. Exhale, bring them together in front of your chest. Repeat three to five times.

6. Breathing counts: Silently count with the breath, inhaling and exhaling through the nostrils (optional: hand on your belly).

   a. Inhale 1, 2, 3.

   b. Exhale 1, 2, 3.

   c. Repeat three times.

7. Standing breathing flow: Coordinate the motions with the breath. To slow the pace, breathe in and out (or out and in) in each position. (Sequence may be done seated.)

   • Tree Hands: Bring the palms together, fingers pointed up, thumbs to the sternum. Inhale, exhale in position.

   • Tree Breathing: Keep the palms together as they move.

      a. Inhale and reach the hands up.

      b. Exhale hands back down.

      c. Repeat two or three times.

   • Half Moon, One Arm

      a. Raise the right arm overhead with an inhalation.

      b. Exhale and lean left.

      c. Inhale back to center.

      d. Exhale, lowering the right arm.

      e. Repeat with the left arm and continue, swaying from side to side with the breath.

   • Tree Breathing: Repeat two to three times

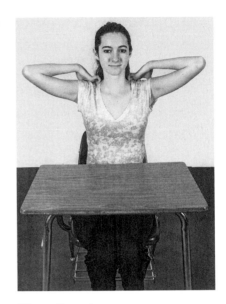

Elbow Pumping

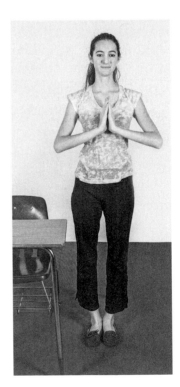

Tree Hands

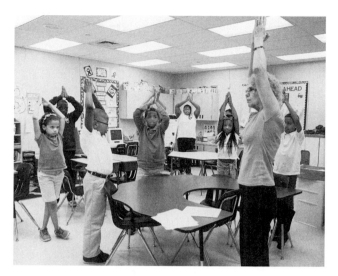

Tree Breathing

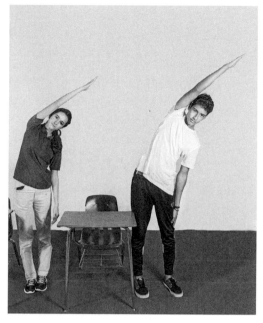

Half Moon One Arm

8. Huh Breath three times: Use to start and end each lesson (standing or seated).
   a. Inhaling, shrug your shoulders up toward your ears.
   b. Exhaling, drop them down with a "huh."

Please note that multi-posture flows such as Lesson 7 above appear throughout the curriculum. You may use the full sequence or select individual postures for 1-minute breaks.

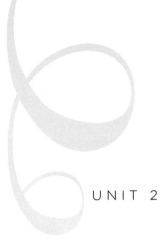

UNIT 2

Relaxation

RELAXATION IS A skill that can be improved with regular practice, just like multiplication or riding a bicycle. Learning to combine breath, posture, and mental focus can improve the ability to self-regulate. Yoga, as we've seen, is a system uniquely designed to promote inner calm.

Moving with focused awareness has a soothing effect on the nervous system. Postures that tuck the chin into the throat notch (Cole, 2008) or press gently on the orbits of the eyes (Robin, 2009) trigger the calming centers of the brain. Forward bending tends to slow respiration; gentle stretching reduces overall tension.

Relaxation is also "an activity of the mind," explains my friend and longtime yoga teacher JoAnn Evans. "It's not something that just happens to you. It's something that you *do*. Only the focused mind can relax. The scattered, agitated mind, skipping from thought to thought, is incapable of relaxing" (personal communication, June 2011).

Through breathing, posture, and mindful awareness practices, this unit will hone your students' relaxation skills.

Practice 1: Your Special Place

Where do you go to relax, free from electronics or other distractions? Do you like to hike in the woods, take a walk down a quiet street, watch the sunset while sitting outside? Imagine that you could go to the most beautiful, peaceful place in the world. It might be a natural setting, in the mountains, in a cave, or by the sea. It could be somewhere no one has ever been before, in outer space, in the center of the earth, or under the ocean. There are no rules, except that this place is very safe and very comfortable. You would feel secure and happy there.

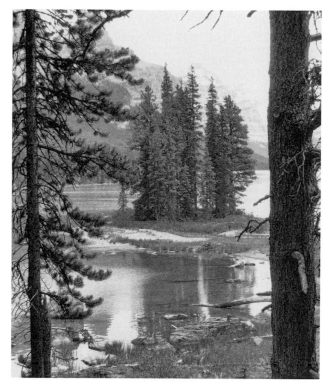
Special Place

Create your special place, by drawing, writing, or making a model. You may keep it private, or share it with the class. (This exercise has also been abbreviated as a Relaxation lesson below.)

Practice 2: Music for Relaxation

Select a song or musical score that creates an atmosphere for relaxation. You may make up your own song or music, or choose from an artist whose work you find calming.

Relaxation Lessons

1. Huh Breath three times
   a. Inhaling, shrug your shoulders up toward your ears.
   b. Exhaling, drop them down with a "huh."
2. Slowing Down Counting Breath: When we increase the duration of the

exhalation, the nervous system is soothed. However, if there's tension or effort in the breath, we don't get the benefits.

Exhale only as long as your body is comfortable, no matter what the count. Silently count with your breath, inhaling and exhaling through the nostrils.

Inhale 1, 2

Exhale 1, 2

Inhale 1, 2

Exhale 1, 2, 3

Inhale 1, 2

Exhale 1, 2, 3

Inhale 1, 2

Exhale 1, 2, 3, 4

Inhale 1, 2

Exhale 1, 2, 3, 4 (Repeat or return to a count that is more comfortable for you.)

3. Calming posture flow seated
   • Huh Breath
   • Bellows Breath 1: Head rest (extended neck).
     a. Interlace your fingers and place your hands behind your head.
     b. Open your elbows wide and look up toward the ceiling.
     c. Rest your head against your hands for three breaths.

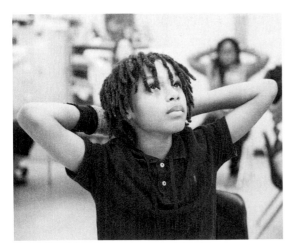

Bellows Breath 1 Head Rest

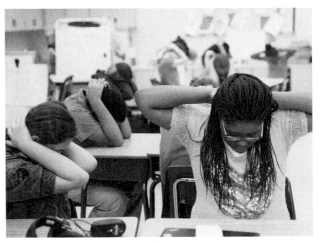

Bellows Breath 2 Chin Tuck

- Bellows Breath 2: Chin tuck (neck flexed).
  a. With your fingers interlaced behind your head, tuck your chin down toward your throat.
  b. Rest your hands against your head for three breaths.
- Bellows Lean
  a. Keep your fingers interlaced behind your head, facing forward.
  b. Lean left; lean right.
- Bellows Breath 2: Chin tuck (neck flexed). Repeat for another breath.
- Palm Stretch
  a. Interlace your fingers and turn the palms out straight in front of you.
  b. Elevate the arms overhead with the palms facing out.
- Palm Stretch and Lean
  a. Use Palm Stretch hand position with your arms stretched overhead.
  b. Lean right; lean left.

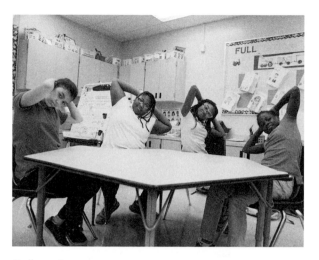

Bellows Lean

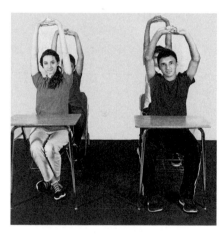

Palm Stretch

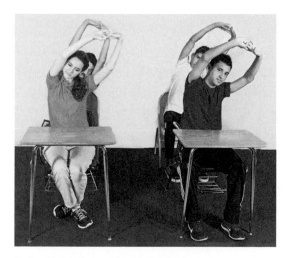

Palm Stretch and Lean Seated

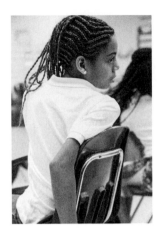

Pretzel Twist

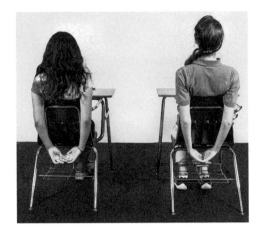

Chair Half Fish

- Seated Pretzel Twist
    a. Bring your left hand across the body and reach for the right side of the chair seat.
    b. Bring the right arm over the back of the chair.
    c. Twist to the right. Reverse hand positions and twist left.
- Chair Half Fish: Reach your arms over the back of the chair and interlace your fingers. (You may reach the hands behind your back if that is more comfortable.)
- Bellows Breath 2: Chin tuck (neck flexed) for three breaths.
4. Calming Sequence standing (variation of the above routine implemented by Sondra Sellitti with two high school classes in spring 2015).
    - Huh Breath
    - Bellows Breath 1: Head rest (extended neck).
        a. Interlace your fingers and place your hands behind your head.
        b. Open your elbows wide and look up toward the ceiling.
        c. Rest your head against your hands for three breaths.
    - Bellows Breath 2: Chin tuck (neck flexed).
        a. From Bellows 1, tuck your chin down toward your throat.
        b. Relax your elbows and rest your hands against your head for three breaths.
    - Bellows Lean
        a. With your fingers interlaced behind your head, lean left.
        b. Reverse.

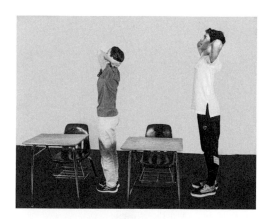

Bellows Breath 1 Head Rest Standing

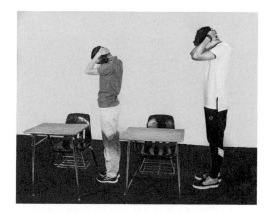

Bellows Breath 2 Chin Tuck Standing

- Bellows Breath 2: Chin tuck (neck flexed) for another breath.
- Palm Stretch
  a. Interlace your fingers and turn the palms out.
  b. Extend the elbows and wrists away from the body straight in front of you.
- Palm Stretch and Lean
  a. Use Palm Stretch hand position with your arms stretched overhead.
  b. Lean right; lean left.

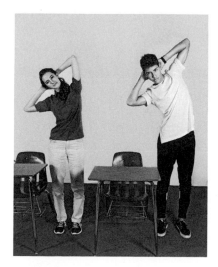

Bellows Lean

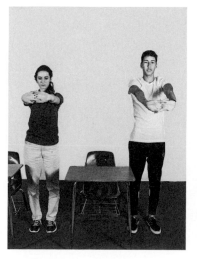

Palm Stretch Front

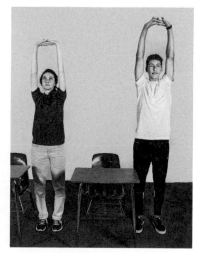

Palm Stretch Upward

- Pretzel Twist
  a. Bring the hands to the hips.
  b. Twist to the right and look over the right shoulder.
  c. Still in position, look over the left shoulder.
  d. Twist to the left and look left.
  e. Still in position, look over the right shoulder.
  f. Repeat both sides.
- Umbrella Squeeze
  a. Clasp the hands behind your back. If this is uncomfortable, place the hands on the hips and skip c.
  b. Gently squeeze the shoulder blades together.
  c. Elevate the arms gently; release.
  - Bellows Breath 2: Chin tuck (neck flexed) for three breaths.
5. Tense and Relax seated: This mindful awareness practice is a variation of progressive muscle relaxation.
  a. Shrug your shoulders toward your ears; drop and relax.

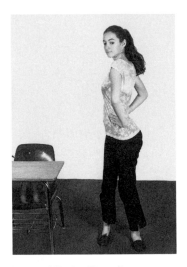

Pretzel Twist Standing

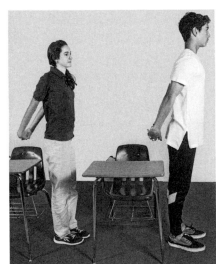

Umbrella Squeeze

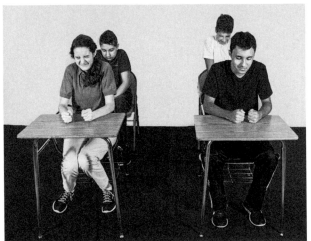

Progressive Muscle Relaxation

b. Raise your right arm out to your side and make a tight fist. Tense. Drop and relax.

c. Raise your left arm out to your side and make a tight fist. Tense. Drop and relax.

d. Tense and squeeze your facial muscles; relax.

e. Squeeze your shoulder blades together in back. Release and relax.

f. Tighten your belly muscles. Release and relax.

g. Raise your right foot an inch off the floor. Drop and relax.

h. Raise your left foot an inch off the floor. Drop and relax.

i. Tense your toes. Release and relax.

j. Tense your whole body.

k. Release and gently shake out your arms and legs.

l. Soft Belly Breaths three times.

6. Visualization Relaxation: Your Special Place. Take a moment to imagine that you could go to the most beautiful, peaceful place in the world—your special place—in the mountains or by the sea, or somewhere that no one has ever been before, somewhere peaceful and safe, where you feel secure and happy. This is your special place, where only you can go. Take three slow deep belly breaths while you rest in your special place. When you are ready, open your eyes.

7. Guided Relaxation: Floating on a Cloud (Goldberg, 2004b).

   Sit comfortably at your desk. Stack your one fist atop the other, and let your forehead rest on your hands. Or choose another position that feels good to you.

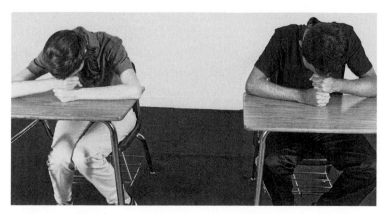

Guided Relaxation

Take a moment to get really comfortable in your seat (pause).

Now it's time to float on an imaginary cloud, one that's soft and fluffy, and made especially for you. It's just your size, strong enough to support you completely, and so soft that it's like resting on cotton balls.

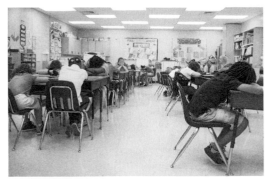

Cloud

This cloud fits your body perfectly; you feel completely safe and secure. Imagine floating in the sky with the birds, so peaceful, so quiet. Your breathing is as soft as the sound of a gentle breeze. You are completely supported, so you can let go all effort. Let go all worry. You are safe and comfortable and secure. Feel the tension melting away from your face and shoulders like ice melting in the warm sun.

Breathe in (pause); breathe out (pause); Breathe in, breathe out. Notice how relaxed your legs have become. Breathe in (pause); breathe out (pause). Notice how relaxed your arms have become. Breathe in (pause); breathe out (pause). Notice how relaxed your forehead and jaws have become, your cheeks, your eyes. Feel your whole body relax. Breathe in (pause); breathe out (pause).

Feel your body very calm, very still. This is how it feels to be relaxed: comfortable, peaceful, safe. The next time someone tells you to relax, remember this feeling: comfortable, peaceful, safe. This is relaxation (pause).

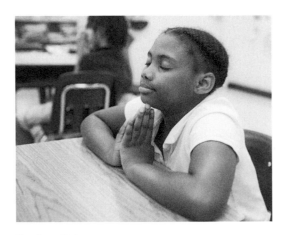

Feeling Calm

Now it's time to float your cloud back down to the ground. Begin to wiggle your toes and fingers. Feel your feet like roots working into the earth. Stretch your fingers and toes, your arms and legs; yawn, as if you were awakening from a long nap. Take another moment to center yourself, breathing in, and breathing out. Rub your palms together and feel the warmth in your palms. Slowly open your eyes. Notice how calm and peaceful you feel.

8. Huh Breath three times
    a. Inhaling, shrug your shoulders up toward your ears.
    b. Exhaling, drop them down with a "huh."

Note that you may select from the preceding relaxation exercises to supplement subsequent units. For example, Your Special Place fits well as an addition to the units on Exercise and Expressing. You may include Music for Relaxation with any lesson. A minute of Slowing Down Counting Breaths may be added to the Intention unit, before tests. If your students especially enjoy Floating on a Cloud, use it as a go-to relaxation lesson whenever you have a few extra minutes at the end of class.

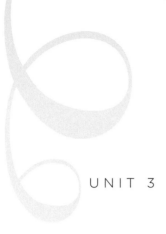

UNIT 3

Exercise

EXERCISE CHANGES THE shape and tone of the body. It also alters the patterns of heartbeat and respiration, affecting how you feel physically and mentally. Exercise-induced stress, which brings about shifts in the nervous system, is very different from the stress of frustration or anxiety (Selye, 1974)—it feels good. As discussed in Chapter 11, exercise also enhances learning readiness and executive function.

In the BREATHE FIRST curriculum, lessons include the elements of strength, flexibility, and balance.

Strength

Muscle strength increases endurance and resilience and is essential for sitting and standing erect. Standing up straight and tall contribute to feeling more powerful and self-assured. Feeling strong in a posture spills over into many aspects of a student's life. People who move with greater ease and confidence are less likely targets for bullying.

Strength and stamina begin with the body but go beyond the physical. Inner strength builds the confidence to speak one's mind and trust one's judgment. Knowing how to stand upright helps students stand up for themselves in inter-personal encounters.

Flexibility

Forced stretching activates the stretch reflex, causing resistance and increased muscle tension. Nothing is forced in yoga. Rather, yoga breaks enhance flexibility through slow steady holding and breathing in postures.

Increased agility facilitates movement in all forms of exercise, as well as standing and sitting. Through the release of muscle tension, students experience a greater openness in their bodies. A more supple body leads to an inner soften-ing. This has been demonstrated by the many examples of changes in students' responses to themselves and others after practicing yoga.

As the body becomes more flexible, it is easier to relax; as the body relaxes, the mind follows.

Balance

Yoga is a system that balances the whole body. It works both sides of the body equally, so that opposing muscle groups are both strengthened and stretched. This also stabilizes joints. Postures move the spine in six directions, with forward and back bending, rotation to each side, and lateral flexion (side bending) to both sides.

Balance postures, like other complex motor movements, exercise the cere-bellum, the portion of the brain that coordinates speech, thinking, attention, feelings, and social skills; this type of exercise strengthens the neural connec-tions involved in many important cognitive functions (Ratey, 2008).

Stability in balance combines strength and flexibility. Standing on one foot builds strong bones and joints. Making the tiny adjustments to maintain balance in the standing ankle requires flexibility in the joints; it improves proprioception—awareness of one's position in motion and stillness. These practices require one-pointed focus, refining a student's capacity to attend.

Practice 1: Posture and Perspective

This practice can be a discussion or journal assignment.

1. Observe how others stand and move. Consider a celebrity, an athlete, and/or a political figure. What assumptions do you make based on what you see? Whether these are right or wrong, how does it affect your view of these individuals? Give specific examples.
2. Can you change how others perceive you by the way you stand and move? Try it and describe the effect (for more on this concept, see Unit 11).
3. Does shifting your physical posture alter how you view yourself? How you feel? Try it and describe the effect (see Posture and breathing, Lesson 2 below).

Practice 2: Exercise Journal

How much time do you spend moving each day? Keep a daily log of the amount of time that you spend walking, bicycling, doing yoga, dancing, playing sports, or other forms of exercise for one week.

1. Type of movement
2. Duration
3. How you felt during exercise
4. How you felt after exercise

Practice 3: Breathing Rhythm

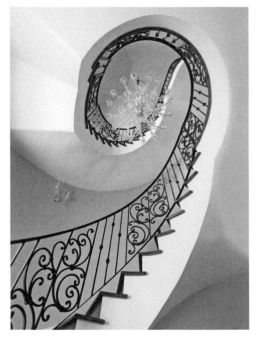
Breathing Stairwell

The breath flows in and out, in a rhythm. Sometimes we breathe quickly, when we are running or exercising. Sometimes we breathe slowly, when we are resting or sitting quietly. Illustrate the rhythm of your breathing when you are moving quickly, and when you are at rest. You may use a line graph or a bell curve.

Or it may look like a spiraling staircase that you walk up and down. This is your breathing rhythm, so use a visual format that is meaningful to you.

Exercise Lessons

1. Huh Breath three times
2. Posture and breathing
   • Grounded Sitting: Angles and lines.

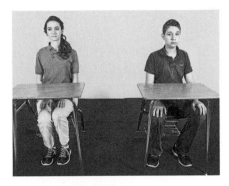

   a. Plant your feet firmly on the ground.
   b. How many 90-degree angles can you form in your body: Knees? Hips?
   c. How many straight lines: neck, back, hips to knees, knees to ankles?

   Observe your breathing in this posture. How does it feel?

Grounded Sitting

   • Slumped Sitting

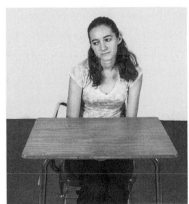

   d. Now let your back round and your shoulders slump.
   e. Hang your head forward.

   Observe your breathing in this posture. Is it more difficult to take a deep breath? How does it feel?

   • Grounded Sitting: Angles and lines. Return to an upright, straight seated posture. How does this change your breathing? How does it make you feel?

Slumped

3. Three-Part Breath: When you exercise, you breathe in different ways. You've practiced soft belly breathing, which enhances relaxation. Now we'll practice using your diaphragm more fully, increasing the movement of the breath throughout your rib and chest area. (All breathing is through the nostrils)
   a. Inhale and softly fill your belly.
   b. Exhale, as the belly gently relaxes.
   c. Inhale and softly fill your belly and feel the breath widening your rib cage.

d. Exhale and gently release the breath from the belly and rib cage.

e. Inhale and softly fill your belly, widen your rib cage, and feel the breath open your chest.

f. Exhale and gently release the breath from the belly, rib cage, and chest. (Repeat e and f twice more.)

g. Inhale and softly fill your belly.

h. Exhale, as the belly gently relaxes.

4. Standing Strength series

a. Chair: Stand with your feet hip distance apart, hands at your hips. Slide your hands down your thighs as you bend your knees as if you were sitting on a stool. For an additional challenge, inhale and raise your arms up alongside your ears. Breathe in the pose.

b. Desk Warrior 1: Stand behind your desk, with your hip and fingertips touching the chair for support. Step one foot forward, bending the forward knee. Elevate the non-supporting arm. Stand straight and tall. Step back and repeat with the opposite foot forward.

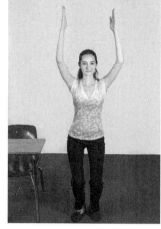

Chair

c. Warrior 1 back bend: From Warrior 1, clasp your hands behind your back and lift the chest. Gaze at the ceiling or wall in front of you, without dropping your head back. Repeat with the opposite leg forward.

d. Shake it out: Fling your arms and hands, jiggle your legs, release your neck and shoulders.

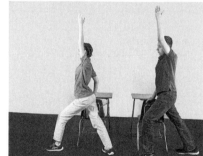

Desk Warrior

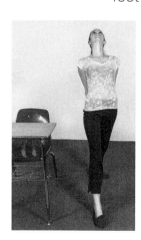

Warrior 1 Back Bend

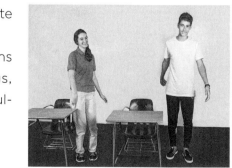

Shake It Out

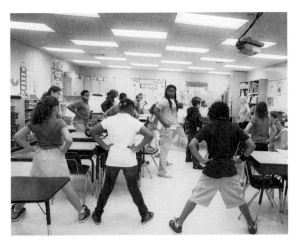

Warrior Stance

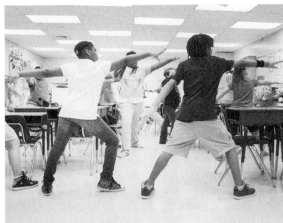

Warrior

e. Warrior 2 stance: Stand with your feet wide apart and your hands on your hips. Feel your strength.

f. Warrior 2: From the previous pose, turn your toes to the right. Bend your right knee and stretch your arms out to the sides. Turn your head to look past your right fingertips. Repeat on the left.

g. Shake it out: Shake all the tension out of your arms and legs.

5. Standing Flexibility series

a. Chair Down Dog: Stand facing the back of your chair with your hands draped over the top. Begin to walk backward away from the chair, feeling the stretch in your back. Look at the floor without dropping your head. Keep your feet under your hips and your hands on the chair. Breathe. Walk your feet forward to release the pose.

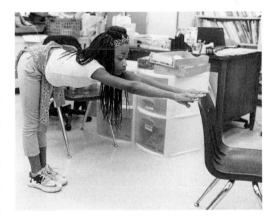

Chair Down Dog

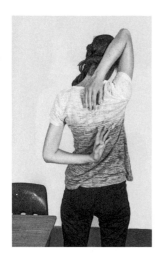

Cow's Head Arms

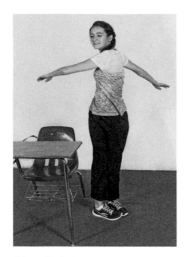

Slow Twister

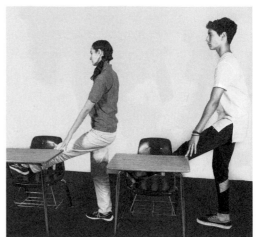

Chair Calf Stretch

b. Cow's Head arm stretch: Standing upright, reach up high with your right arm. Bend the elbow and reach your palm down your back. Reach behind your back with the left arm, bringing your fingertips close to your other hand. Don't force the stretch. Relax and breathe. Repeat on the other side.

c. Slow Twister: Stand with your arms at your sides. Slowly twist from side to side, letting your arms swing freely.

d. Chair Calf Stretch: Holding the chair with at least one hand, slide your heel onto the seat. Feel the stretch without force. Step down and repeat with the other leg.

e. Rag Doll: Stand facing away from your chair. Being certain that you have space for your head, place your hands on your thighs and soften your knees. Let your arms lead as you hang gently forward toward the ground. Do not hang down if you have high blood pressure, heart disease, or seizure disorder, or if it just doesn't feel right. Avoid immediately after eating.

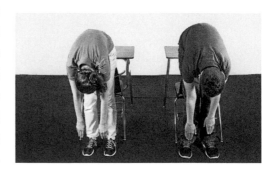

Rag Doll

6. Standing Balance series. Use your eyes to establish a focal point by fixing your gaze about your height in front of you on the ground. Keep your breathing slow and steady. For some students, a visual cue for the eyes makes balance more accessible.

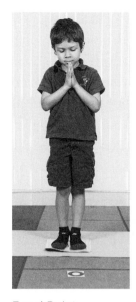
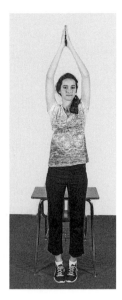

Focal Point   Tall Tree

a. Tall Tree Flow: Stand in front of your desk in Tree Hands, palms together. Inhale and raise both arms over your head. Exhale in the pose. With the next inhalation, come up on your toes. Exhale and lower your heels. Inhale as you rise up on your toes, and exhale down on your heels. Repeat. Inhale in position; exhaling, float the hands back down in front of your chest.

b. Tall Tree Hold: This time stand with one hand on your desk or chair. Inhale and elevate the heels. Exhale in the pose, heels still lifted. If you are comfortable, take two more deep breaths in the pose, remaining up on your toes. Elevate your arms overhead, palms together, and hold the position on your toes for one more breath. Slowly lower. (You may follow this pose with Chair Calf Stretch, 5d.)

c. Tree Prep 1: Toe Stand. Stand with one hand on your desk or chair. Bring your weight onto your right foot and raise your left heel off the ground. Place your foot back down and switch to the other side.

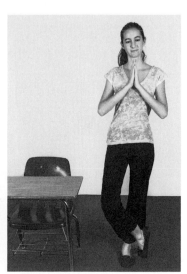

d. Tree Prep 2: Toe Cross. With your weight on your left foot, reach your right toes across your left foot in front. Breathe and bring the palms together at your chest. Step down and reverse.

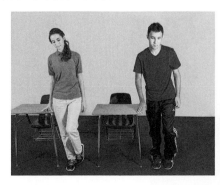

Toe Stand

Toe Cross

e. Standing Crane: Standing on both feet, find a focal point for your eyes. Shift the weight to the right foot. Relax the wrists and breathe. Slowly raise your left leg, bending the knee. Lower and repeat on the other side.

7. Eye exercises: Tiny muscles in the eyes control movement in all directions. It's important to exercise and rest your eyes. Sit up comfortably in your seat, with soft belly breathing.

a. Up/down: Without moving your head, look up with your eyes; look down. Repeat twice more.

b. Rest with the eyes closed

c. Side to side: Without moving your head, look right and left three times. Rest.

d. Diagonal: Stretch your eyes to the upper right and lower left three times. Rest. Now stretch your eyes to the upper left and lower right three times. Rest.

e. Eye palming: Rub your palms together to make them warm. Cup the warm palms over the closed eyes to block out all the light. Breathe in and out, soft belly breaths, three times.

8. Huh Breaths three times.

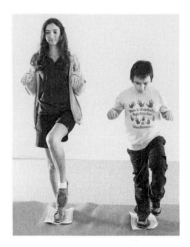

Crane Balance

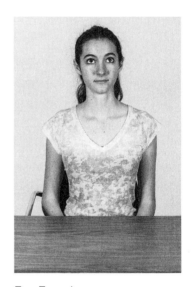

Eye Exercises

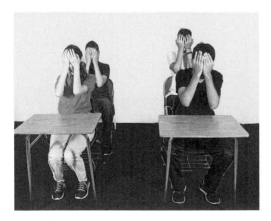

Eye Palming

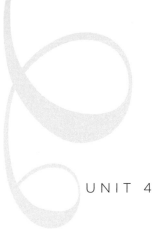

UNIT 4

Attention

ATTENTION IS FOCUSED awareness. It involves listening and observing without judging or anticipating. These are mindful practices.

Have you ever heard an account from two different people who had witnessed the same incident at the same time from the same vantage point, yet each had a different description of the event? Even when they are certain that their perceptions accurately reflect the facts, what people see is often colored by their own experience and assumptions. Instead of paying attention to what is, they inadvertently fill in the blanks based on what they expect.

Researchers Simons and Chabris conducted an experiment in 1999 that revealed a great deal about paying attention. While watching a video of students tossing basketballs, subjects were asked to count the number of passes between specific players. Half of the subjects were so focused on counting the passes that they missed a gorilla walking across the scene, thumping its chest. When I watched the video the first time, I missed it, too. I didn't believe it until I viewed it again and saw the gorilla for myself.

This phenomenon, according to the study authors, is an example of selective attention, which occurs when people's focus is so narrow that they miss something significant occurring right in front of them. "This experiment reveals two things: that we are missing a lot of what goes on around us, and that we have no idea that we are missing so much" (Simons & Chabris, 2010). The Selective Attention Test and the Monkey Business Illusion can be viewed at the Invisible Gorilla (www.theinvisiblegorilla.com).

An important distinction between yoga and other forms of exercise is this quality of attention. You can run on a treadmill while watching TV or talking on the phone and still get a good workout. With yoga, however, the mind is as engaged as the body. As you may recall from Chapter 16, when you tried to balance on one foot while reading a text, it was really difficult. You have to pay attention.

Yoga also employs bilateral movements. Postures that cross one arm or leg over the other are effective for "turning on" the brain (Dennison & Dennison, 1986) and enhancing a student's capacity to focus. Twisting postures where limbs cross the midline of the body serve a similar function.

Yoga requires presence and encourages an open, inquiring mind. An ideal place to practice paying attention is within your own body. By noticing your breathing, how your body feels in movement and stillness, and the activity of your own mind, you become more skillful in the art of focused awareness.

Practice 1: What Do You See?

Show the Monkey Business Illusion to your students and explore the concept of selective attention. Ask them to discuss or write about experiences that they have missed by focusing too much on one thing (such as texting or playing computer games) to the exclusion of others.

Practice 2: What Catches Your Attention?

a. Make a list of things and people that you do pay attention to.

b. Make a list of things and people that you do not pay attention to.

c. In small groups, compare and discuss the lists.

Practice 3: Attention Journal

For one week, experiment with paying close attention.

1. Note what happens when you really pay attention to a conversation with a friend.
2. Give your full attention to a movie or television show.
3. Eat a meal with awareness of every bite.

Describe how these experiences differ from your habitual patterns.

Attention Lessons

1. Huh Breath three times
2. Pause breathing inhalation: 1–2-minute practice. Divide the in-breath into three parts.

   a. Inhale, pause; inhale, pause; complete the inhalation.

   b. Exhale fully.

   c. Take a natural inhalation and exhalation.

   d. Repeat a–c.

   When you finish, sit and take three additional deep breaths. Notice if the duration of your inhalation has changed.

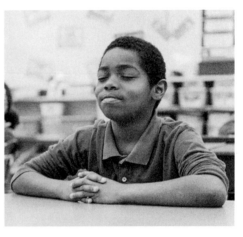

Attention to Breathing

3. Pause breathing exhalation: 1–2-minute practice. Divide the out-breath into three parts.

   a. Take a natural inhalation.

   b. Exhale, pause; exhale, pause; complete the exhalation.

   c. Take a natural inhalation and exhalation.

   d. Repeat a–c.

   When you finish, sit and take three additional deep breaths. Notice if the length of your inhalation or exhalation has changed.

4. Simply Notice (courtesy Steven Templin, www.stevetemplin.com). Here are a few suggestions for simply noticing (10 seconds at a time is helpful):

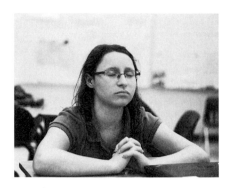

Simply Notice

a. You can notice the sensations in your feet . . . just be curious . . . and take a gentle breath.

b. You can notice a sound or two in your present environment . . . notice curiously . . . and breathe.

c. Breathe: Gentle, slow breathing gives you something to notice while balancing your nervous system.

d. Notice the thoughts in your head and how they make you feel . . . and breathe.

e. Notice something for which you are grateful . . . appreciate the feel of it . . . and breathe.

5. Seated Attention sequence

• Elbows

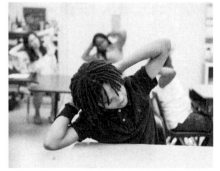

Elbow Lean

a. Elbow lean: Place one hand on each shoulder as you inhale. Exhale and lean to the right. Inhale upright. Exhale and lean to the left. Repeat.

b. Elbow circles: With one hand on each shoulder, circle the elbows in one direction. Reverse. This time make the circles larger. Now smaller.

c. Elbow twist: With the hands on the shoulders, twist your body to the right; then to the left. Repeat.

d. Elbow pumping (see photo p. 176): Inhale in position. Exhale and bring your elbows together in front. Inhale and bring your elbows toward one another in back.

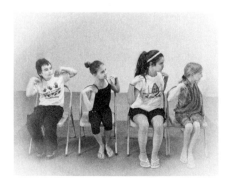

Elbow Twist

- Seated Eagle Arms: Cross the right arm over the left at the elbow. Now cross the wrists or bring the backs of the palms together. This is the beak of your eagle. Release and switch to the left arm on top.

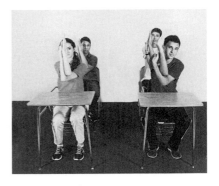

Seated Eagle Arms

- Palm Stretch (see photo p. 181): Thread your fingers together. Turn your hands inside out by pressing your palms away from you. Release and rethread your fingers with the opposite thumb on top. Repeat the stretch.
- Half Lotus: Cross your right foot over your left thigh. If this is not comfortable or your clothing makes this awkward, cross at the ankle or shin. Bring your palms together in Tree Hands. Inhale and elevate the hands. Exhale and lower. Release and sit with both feet on the floor. Repeat with your left foot.

6. Standing Eagle 1: Cross your right arm over the left at the elbow. Then bring the palms or backs of the hands together. Cross your left foot over your right ankle, touching the toes or foot to the floor for stability.

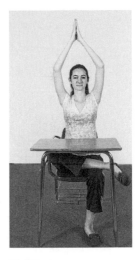

7. Walking Meditation: Silently walk around the classroom and notice how your body moves and how it feels.

a. Are your arms still or do they swing when you walk?

b. Do your hands move or rest close to your sides?

Half Lotus

c. Do you step on your whole foot at one time, roll from heel to toe, or do something in-between?

d. How does it feel to step in different ways?

e. Are there parts of your body that don't move much when you walk? Parts that move a lot?

f. What do you notice about your breathing when you walk?

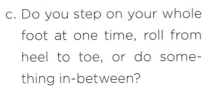

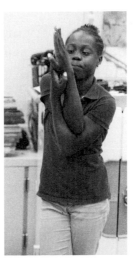

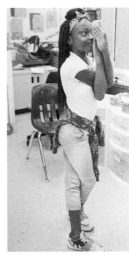

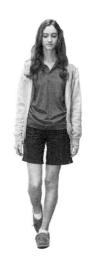

Eagle Arms   Eagle Standing   Walking Meditation

8. Focusing practice (seated; adapted with permission from the 31 Points Exercise by Swami Rama of the Himalayan Institute (Rama, 1982, pp. 110–111).

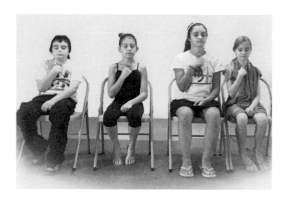

Focusing Practice

Paying attention to one point at a time is an effective tool for improving focus. In the classic 31 Points Exercise taught at the Himalayan Institute, there is no touch—the process of focused attention is entirely mental; the points are slightly different; and it's practiced while relaxing lying down.

To facilitate this exercise for classroom use, students will sit up and use a light touch. They will begin using the left forefinger; then will switch to the right. In time, it may be practiced as originally intended, directing the mind to each point without touching them.

This sequence will take about a minute. To extend this exercise for 2 to 5 minutes, students breathe in and out one time (or more) at each point before moving on to the next.

Before you begin, be sure that the students are familiar with each of the areas of the body that you will be naming. (For foreign language study, name each part in that language.)

Instructions: Sit up comfortably straight in your chair. Focus on soft belly breathing. To begin, use your left forefinger to very lightly touch each of the following points, as I name them.

1. Between the eyebrows
2. Throat notch (base of the throat)
3. Right shoulder joint
4. Right inner elbow
5. Right inner wrist
6. The tip of each finger starting with right thumb
7. Right forefinger
8. Right middle finger
9. Right ring finger

10. Right pinkie finger
11. Right inner wrist
12. Right inner elbow
13. Right shoulder joint outside
14. Right shoulder joint inside
15. Throat notch
    Change hands: Use the right forefinger to lightly touch:
16. Left shoulder joint
17. Left inner elbow
18. Left inner wrist
19. The tip of each finger starting with left thumb
20. Left forefinger
21. Left middle finger
22. Left ring finger
23. Left pinkie finger
24. Left inner wrist
25. Left inner elbow
26. Left shoulder joint outside
27. Left shoulder joint inside
28. Throat notch
29. Sternum
30. Throat notch
31. Between the eyes
    Now rest with palms upturned in your lap, one atop the other, touching the thumb tips lightly. Pay attention to your breathing.
9. Huh Breath three times

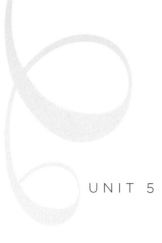

Tuning In and Tuning Out

MOST ADOLESCENTS ARE leading virtual lives, tuned in to electronics, but tuned out from what may be happening in real time. According to a Kaiser Foundation study, teens typically use media content for 7 to 10 hours per day (Rideout, Foehr, & Roberts, 2010). While these distractions may provide a break from the pressure of schoolwork and other people, they also create distance.

Music blasting from ear buds drowns out the world around them. Video games can become a substitute for direct interaction with others. Some teens tune out in these ways to blunt unpleasant feelings and avoid sources of conflict, inhibiting true social engagement.

Concern with physical appearance, what others say and do, and social drama consume a great deal of adolescents' attention. Cars, sex, and the quest for popularity also preoccupy much of their time. Although different from electronics, such activities create an outward focus—another form of tuning out.

Tuning in, on the other hand, is the process of increasing awareness and connection—the antecedent to empathy. It requires acknowledging one's feelings and engaging in the messy task of figuring out how to get along with others. The ability to make genuine connections begins with self-awareness. Deepening relationships with others often necessitates self-reflection.

What we tune in to also has a tremendous impact on our well-being. Many experts believe that laughter and positive thoughts promote healing (Cousins, 1979; Thoms, 2011). In contrast, worry and anxiety interfere with the ability to think clearly and wreak havoc with the immune system (McEwen, 2002). Despite the importance of controlling the direction of the thoughts, it's not easy to do. Tuning out distractions requires a highly disciplined mind, while tuning in to the chosen focal point requires consistent practice.

Practice 1: Musical Listening

Listen carefully to an orchestral or other musical arrangement. Can you identify some of the instruments and the parts that they are playing?

Practice 2: Outside Sensations

Outside walking or sitting, tune in to the sounds, sights, and movement around you—animals, wind, trees, sun. Write a description of what you experience when you tune in to the natural world.

Practice 3: Tuning In to What?

What activities are so engrossing for you that you tune in completely and tune out the distractions around you? How many different types of activities create this response among your classmates and friends: movement, music, reading, watching?

1. Poll friends, classmates, and family members.
2. Make a chart or graph with the varied responses.

Categorize the activities:

1. Electronic device required or not
2. Movement involved or stationary
3. Done alone or with others

4. Costs money or free

5. Silent or sound

Practice 4: Tuning In Journal

In the next week, complete four tuning in practices. Choose at least one tuning in activity that does not involve electronics, is free of cost, involves movement, and that you do alone. Practice another that meets the same criteria but is done with others. Practice one that is silent and one that involves sounds. You may use exercises that you learn in this unit if you wish. Keep a journal of these experiences.

Tuning In and Tuning Out Lessons

1. Huh Breath three times

2. Humming Breath (seated or standing): This calming breath lengthens the exhalation while you tune in to the sound of the breath.

   a. Close your mouth, keeping a slight space between your top and bottom teeth.

   b. Take a deep breath in through the nose.

   c. Exhaling, quietly hum as you breathe out as long as you can, listening.

   d. Experiment with pitch:

      i. Make the hum slightly higher this time.

      ii. Now hum at a lower pitch.

   Do you feel the vibration in your mouth and face? How do the different pitches feel? Do they affect the duration or quality of the exhalation?

   e. Take another deep breath in. Exhale with the humming sound that you prefer.

3. Ah Ha Breathing, 1 to 5 minute silent practice

   a. Sit quietly, practicing soft belly breathing.

   b. Observe the movement of your belly and the feeling of the breath.

   c. Hear the sound "ah" when you inhale.

   d. Hear the sound "ha" when you exhale.

   e. Each time your mind wanders or is distracted, return your attention to the sound of the breath.

4. Tuned In to Sound
   - Listening
     a. Sit upright and tune in to the sound while the teacher strikes the vibratone, bowl, soft symbols, or chime.
     b. When you no longer hear the sound, raise your hand.
   - Holding sound
     c. Now we'll try again. Listen to the sound while the teacher strikes the vibratone.
     d. This time see how long you can hear that sound in your own head.
     e. When other thoughts and sounds begin to creep in, can you re-create that peaceful sound for yourself?

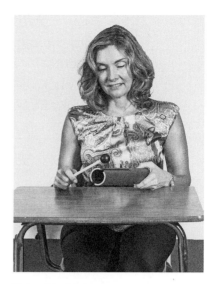

Tuned In Listening

5. Standing Chair Stretching: Slow stretching helps us tune in. Observe your body and breathing in order to stretch without strain, without pain, without force. This requires focus.
   a. Hamstring Stretch: Stand facing your chair seat. Hold the back of the chair or seat as you step one foot onto the near edge of the seat. Gently slide your foot toward the back edge of the seat. If you are comfortable, lean your upper body forward toward your leg. Repeat on the other side.
   b. Chair Windmill: With your hands on the back of your chair, walk backward away from the chair. Keep your feet under your hips and stretch your back

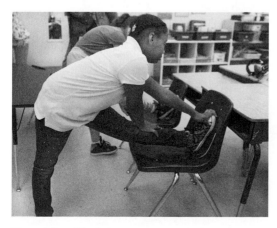

Hamstring Stretch

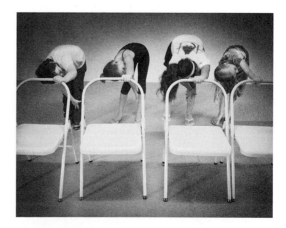

Chair Windmill

in Chair Down Dog. Lower your right hand to the outside of your left thigh or shin. Gently rotate your chest to the left. Come back to Chair Down Dog and repeat on the other side.

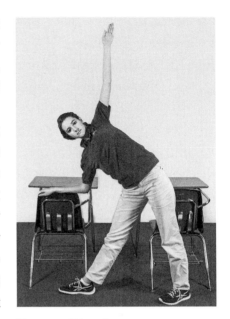

Forearm Triangle

c. Forearm Triangle: Stand with your feet wide apart. Place your right hand on the back of your chair. Turn the toes of both feet to the right. Bending your right elbow, gently lean to the right until your forearm is draped over the back of your chair. (You may also use the desk surface.) Slowly raise the left arm up toward the ceiling, with your chest and back long. Breathe in the pose and notice the openness in your left side. Slowly lower the left arm and push up into standing. Release and reverse.

6. Standing Chair Balance: Balance requires inner focus and steady breathing. Use your gaze to tune in to one spot approximately your height in front of you when balancing.

a. Chair Tree Prep, Toe Touch: Standing on both feet, find a focal point for your eyes. Shift your weight to your right foot. Lightly place your left toes on top of your right foot. Lower and switch sides.

b. Chair Low Tree: Holding on to the back of your chair or desk, find a focal point for your eyes on the ground about your height in front of you. Shift your weight to your right foot and place your left foot against your inner right shin, below your knee. Release and repeat on the other side.

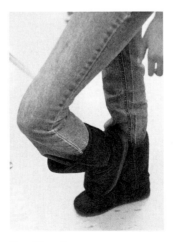

Toe Touch

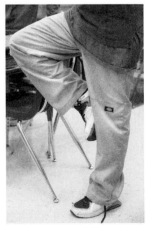

Chair Low Tree

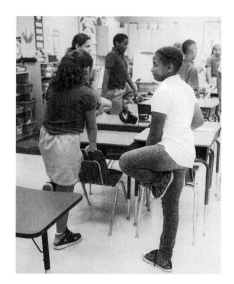

Chair High Tree

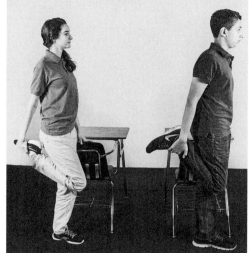

Chair Dancer

c. Chair High Tree: Repeat as above, but if it's comfortable, place your foot above your knee on your inner thigh. (Either below or above the knee works, but don't push directly against the knee.) Keep the breath flowing in and out softly and your gaze on a spot on the floor. Make this silent suggestion: "I am focused; I am calm." Release and repeat on the other side.

d. Chair Dancer: Stand sideways with your left hip near your chair or desk. Hold with the left hand and stand up straight. Breathe in; breathing out, bend your right knee. Reach back for your right ankle or foot. Stand tall with your back long as you breathe in and out. Repeat this silent suggestion: "I am focused; I am calm." Release and repeat on the other side.

7. Turning inward: Withdrawal of the senses. Let's begin turning inward and slowly shutting out distractions.

a. Lightly place your hands over your closed mouth. Notice how easy it is to be quiet in this way.

b. Keep very quiet as you lightly place your hands over your closed eyes. Feel the warmth of your hands as you shut out all the light in this room. If you wish, you may keep your eyes closed as we move on.

c. Lightly cover your ears and close out all of the sound, even my voice.

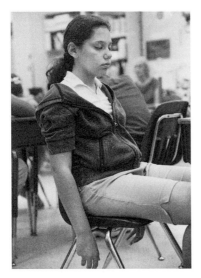

Relaxed Hands

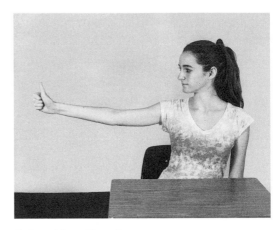

Follow Your Thumb

    d. Now relax your hands at your sides. Take a moment to breathe quietly in this way, and when you are ready, open your eyes.

8. Follow your thumb: Make a soft fist with your thumb outside, pointing upward. Follow your thumb with your eyes as you slowly stretch your arm out to your right side; then to the left. Keep your focus on your thumb as you move it in a slow circle clockwise; then counterclockwise. Release and reverse thumbs.

9. Concentration on a flower
    a. Sit comfortably upright in your seat, feeling your soft belly breathing.
    b. Focus your eyes on the beautiful flower.
    c. Observe the shape of the petals, the variations of the color, the simplicity within the complex arrangement.
    d. Close your eyes and retain the image.
    e. If your mind wanders, open your eyes and return your focus to the flower.

10. Huh Breath three times

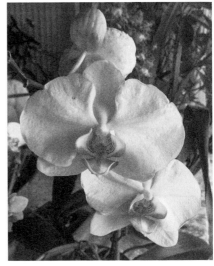

Concentration on a Flower

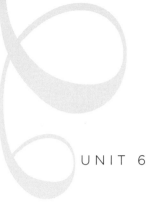

UNIT 6

Heart Opening

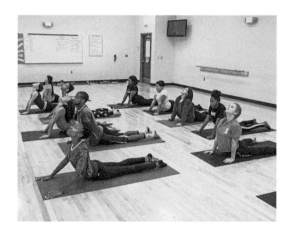

Heart Opening

OURS IS A culture that often encourages a rift between heart and mind. Adults tell teens to "use their heads" and not to "wear their hearts on their sleeves." Certainly, disregarding the intellect is not advisable in decision making. Yet there is a great deal of research that suggests the importance of listening to gut intelligence and heart-based knowledge (Siegel, 2013; Heart Math Institute, 2016).

From hours spent hunched over their computers, self-consciousness about their changing bodies, and the burden of heavy backpacks, many teens habitually slump when standing or sitting. In addition, school and personal stress is at record high levels for teens, resulting in symptoms of depression and fatigue for many adolescents (American Psychological Association, 2014).

When the chest sinks, whether from poor posture or a depressed affect, the respiration is likely to become shallow. As we've seen, breathing and physical posture reflect how a person feels; they also have the capacity to change those feelings. Deepening the breath and opening the heart area through yoga breaks can increase a student's energy level and improve his or her outlook. Practices in gratitude have been shown to enhance physical and emotional health, social success, sleep, empathy, and self-esteem (Morin, 2014).

Caution: Open-hearted postures can be uncomfortable for individuals who are experiencing symptoms of depression. If you observe discomfort or reluctance among your students when they attempt these positions, use the Tuning In pose offered in each sequence instead. You may come back to the full sequence at a later time.

Practice 1: Depression

Research the signs of depression. What are its effects on adolescents? Discuss sources of support in the community for those suffering from depression.

Practice 2: Conflict

Share an experience where your heart and head were in conflict. How did you work out the best course of action?

Practice 3: Language of the Heart

Use four of these terms in sentences or a poem: hard hearted, heartfelt, heart in my mouth, have a heart, take heart, speaking from the heart, heartrending, heartbroken, heart of gold.

Practice 4: Journaling

1. Kindness journal: Each day for one week, perform one act of kindness that you might not customarily do. Record your experiences and feelings.
2. Gratitude journal: List at least five people or things that you are thankful for. Say thank you to at least one person every day for one week. Record your experiences and feelings.

Practice 5: Something I Like About You

1. Students sit or stand in a circle and one student volunteers to go first.
2. Everyone in the class shares (written or oral) one thing that they like about this student. (Requirement: It must be kind, positive, and appropriate for sharing in a group.)
3. Go on to the next volunteer.

With large classes, you may do this practice in small groups (see Chapter 15).

Heart-Opening Lessons

1. Huh Breath three times
2. Warming Breath
   a. Inhale through your nose.
   b. Exhale by letting the breath out slowly through the open, relaxed mouth, as quietly as possible.
   c. Inhale through your nose
   d. Open your mouth, relax it, and exhale into your palm with a slow breath; your palm feels warm.
   e. Repeat twice more.
3. Back-to-Back Partner Breathing
   a. Sit or stand with your back against your partner in a comfortable position.
   b. Begin soft belly breathing through your nose.
   c. After a few moments, notice your partner's breathing. Can you feel her breathing in? Breathing out?
   d. Without forcing your breath in any way, notice if you can match your partner's breathing. Begin your inhalation when she does; begin your exhalation when she does.
   e. If this feels uncomfortable, just go back to observing without changing your own breathing.

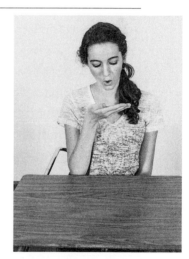

Warming Breath

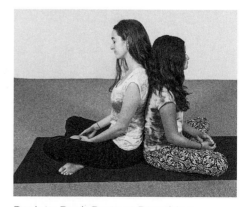

Back to Back Partner Breathing

f. If it feels right, stay with your partner's rhythm until you two, breathing together, become as one.

4. Standing Heart Opening with deep breathing

a. Tree Breathing (Tuning In) (see photo p. 177): Bring the palms together at the chest in Tree Hands. As you breathe in, elevate the hands, keeping your palms together; lower with the exhalation. Repeat.

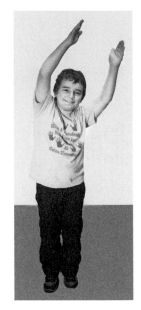

b. Half Moon double arms: Stretch both arms overhead, shoulder distance apart, inhaling. Exhaling, lean left. Inhale back to center. Exhaling, lean right. Repeat twice more with the breath.

c. Shoulder circles (Tuning In): With the arms relaxed at your sides, slowly circle the shoulders in one direction. Use soft belly breathing. Reverse the direction of your circles.

Half Moon Double Arms

d. Umbrella: Begin in Umbrella Squeeze. Clasping or reaching the hands behind your back, gently squeeze the shoulder blades together. Slowly bend forward from the hips, lifting the arms behind you to open your heart. If this is uncomfortable, return to Umbrella Squeeze without clasping the hands.

e. Chair Up Dog: Holding onto the back of your chair with both hands, take a

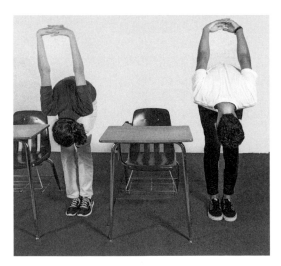

Umbrella

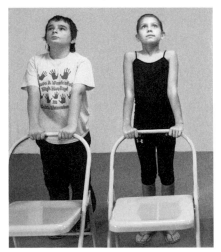

Chair Up Dog

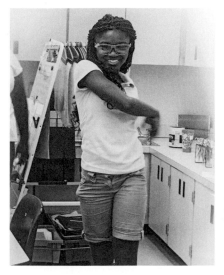

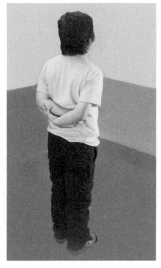

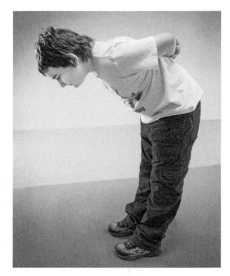

Fast Twister   Half Rag Doll Arms   Half Rag Doll

step back. Activate the muscles in your back and open your chest. Breathing in, look upward, but don't let your head hang back. Exhale. Take another breath in the pose and release with the exhalation.

  f. Fast Twister: Let your arms fly out from your sides as you gently twist from side to side. Pick up some speed. Now slow it down. Notice your breathing.

  g. Half Rag Doll (Tuning In): Stand away from your chair. Clasp your forearms or wrists behind your back. This may be as far as you go today. If you choose, fold forward from the hips, lowering your upper body as far as you are comfortable. (Avoid bending forward if you have high blood pressure, heart disease, seizure disorder, or it just doesn't feel right. Avoid immediately after lunch.)

  h. Tree Breathing (Tuning In) (repeat from above).

5. Bellows Breath Pause
  • Bellows 1: Head rest
    a. Interlace your fingers and place your hands behind your head.
    b. Open your elbows wide and look up toward the ceiling.
    c. Rest your head against your hands.
    d. Take three soft belly breaths in this position.

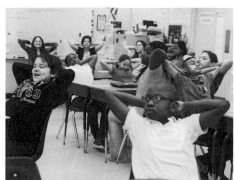

Bellows Breath 1 Head Rest

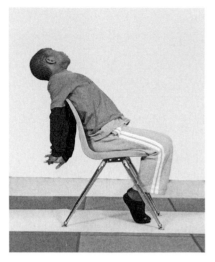

Open Heart Sitting

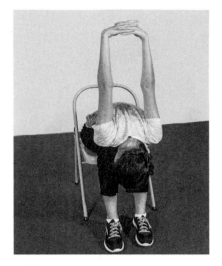

Open Heart Folded Leaf

- Bellows 2: Chin tuck (Tuning In; see photo p. 180)

    e. With your next exhalation, tuck your chin into your chest.

    f. Take three soft belly breaths in this position.

    g. Inhaling, release the hands and let your head float to a neutral position.

6. Seated Heart Opening

    a. Open Heart Sitting: Sit back in your chair and reach your arms around your chair. Clasp your hands or forearms behind your back if it's comfortable for you. Open your chest as you inhale.

    b. Open Heart Folded Leaf: Be certain there is ample room in front of you. Move halfway forward on your chair with your feet securely on the ground and clasp your hands behind your back. Exhaling, fold forward with your hands clasped behind your back in the Open Heart Sitting position. Go only as far as your comfort permits. Release the arms for a Tuning In pose.

    c. Half Fish Open Arms: Sit back in your chair. Drape your arms over the back of your chair if it's comfortable. Take three soft belly breaths.

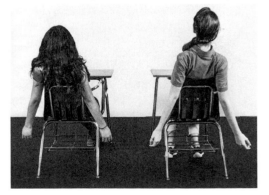

Half Fish Open Arms

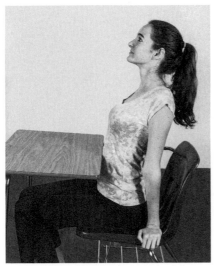
Open Heart Seat Hold

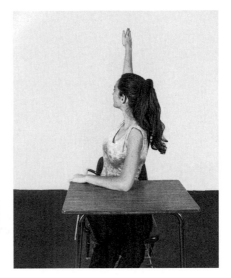
Seated One Arm Twist

    d. Open Heart Seat Hold: Sit upright and hold onto the sides of your seat. Pressing into your hands, gently open your heart, drawing the shoulder blades together in back. Take three soft belly breaths.

    e. Seated One-Arm Twist: Rest your left forearm on your desk. Elevate your right arm alongside your ear. Inhale in position. With an exhalation, slowly twist to the right. Breathe in the posture. With your next exhalation, return to center. Switch sides.

    f. Self-Hug (Tuning In): Reaching your arms across your rib cage, give yourself a huge hug.

7. Gratitude Breathing: Use soft belly breathing.

    a. Hold an image in your mind of something or someone for whom you are grateful.

    b. Inhale, silently saying the word "thank."

    c. Exhale, silently saying the word "you."

    d. Repeat three times.

8. Huh Breath three times

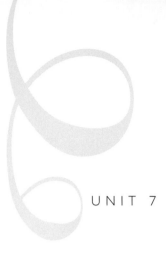

Expressing

ADOLESCENCE IS OFTEN a period of intense emotion. As discussed in Chapter 9, the teen brain is fueled by the "turbo-boosted limbic system" where emotions rule, rather than the prefrontal cortex, where rational decision-making occurs (Giedd, 2015). Anger, fear, and frustration reside closer to the surface in young people, who often have shortened emotional fuses.

Many educators have turned to yoga as a tool for restoring calm after local or national tragedies. Including an element of self-expression within the yoga curriculum offers students an additional outlet for working through painful feelings and releasing anger.

In craniosacral therapy, the mouth, throat, and tongue are described as the "avenue of expression" (Upledger Institute, 2016). This area is the neural highway between the head and the heart. Unexpressed words, thoughts, and emotions are believed to contribute to an energetic bottleneck in the throat area, creating a traffic jam in the transmission of sensory information. In my work as a craniosacral therapist, I find releasing tension from the avenue of expression relieves much discomfort in the jaws, sinuses, neck, shoulders, and lower back. In many cases, emotional and physical release coincide.

Similarly, yoga breathing techniques and postures may be used to open and relax this area. Gentle neck stretches, using sound to open the mouth and throat, and softening the facial muscles serve a function similar to craniosacral massage. Singing vowel sounds extends the exhalation, which also has a calming effect on the nervous system. Removing restrictions from the avenue of expression may prevent mounting frustration and facilitate responsible release of anger and negative emotion.

Practice 1: Emotion Journal

Keep a journal to record your feelings. Notice if your emotions reveal a pattern.

1. Do you feel more easily upset when you are tired or hungry?
2. Do specific activities or individuals provoke more intense feelings than others?
3. Are there activities that change how you feel?
   a. Exercise
   b. Talking to a friend
   c. Listening to music
   d. Eating, drinking water, or resting

Work with one breathing or movement technique that you find calming.

1. Use that technique during or after an emotionally demanding activity.
2. Try it at least once every day for one week.
3. Record the results.

Practice 2: The Three Sieves

Once we say something, it can never be unsaid. There is great power in spoken words.

Sometimes referred to as "The Three Gates," "The Three Sieves" is a story that was included in a text written for educators nearly 100 years ago (Cabot et al., 1918). A sieve is a strainer, similar to a colander that is used to drain the water after cooking pasta. In this story a mother is concerned about her son spreading cruel gossip. She asks him to consider these three questions before repeating a tale that he overheard at school:

1. Is it true?
2. Is it kind?
3. Is it necessary?

In the story, the boy realizes that what he was saying did not pass through these three "sieves" and should not be retold.

For class discussion or written assignment:

1. Describe one incident when you passed your words through one or more of the three sieves before speaking.
2. Did it change what you said? Or not?
3. How did that make you feel?
4. What are the advantages and disadvantages of considering the three sieves before expressing yourself?

Practice 3: Colistening Shoulder to Shoulder

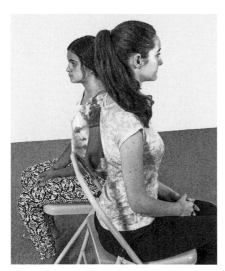

Shoulder to Shoulder Listening

Adapted with permission from the Kripalu Yoga in the Schools Curriculum, 2015. Sit next to your partner at shoulder level, facing opposite directions. Each person has the opportunity to share something of her choosing—a project of interest, a problem she is grappling with, an idea she wants to explore—uninterrupted for 2 minutes. Her partner will listen without revealing any response or reaction—neither words nor expression. After the time is up, the partners switch roles, with the same rules applying.

1. How did it feel to be really listened to?
2. Was it difficult to listen without responding in any way?
3. What did you learn about yourself from this practice?

Practice 4: Colistening Face to Face

Repeat the exercise above, but this time you will sit facing your partner. When you are finished, discuss the experience.

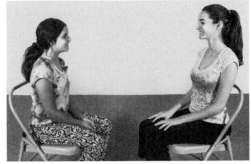

a. Was it more or less difficult to talk and listen while facing your partner?

b. Was it more or less difficult not to respond?

c. How did it feel when you and your partner could interact in a more natural way after the exercise?

d. What did you learn about yourself from this practice?

Face to Face Listening

Expressing Lessons

1. Huh Breath three times
2. Silent Lion Breath
   a. Take a deep breath in and yawn, stretching your mouth open.
   b. Take another deep breath in. Make a tense face: Squeeze your eyes and your mouth and lips closed tightly.
   c. Exhaling, open your mouth and eyes wide without making a sound.
   d. Repeat.
3. Lion Breath (standing or seated): You may use this exercise to consciously release anger or other negative feelings by including discussion before and after.
   a. Take a deep breath in.
   b. Exhaling, silently stretch your tongue down toward your chin, your eyes up toward your scalp, and your fingers out like claws.
   c. Take another deep inhalation, relaxing your face and fingers.
   d. Exhale with a loud roar from deep down in your belly.
   e. Take another deep inhalation.

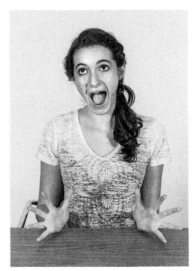

Lion

f. Exhaling, put it all together in Lion Breath: Stretch your tongue down, eyes up, and fingers out, and make a ferocious roar.

g. Close your eyes and breathe normally.

Take a moment to think about something that you wish you had said but never did. Repeat e and f, using the roar to release those unsaid words.

4. Neck Stretches (standing or seated)

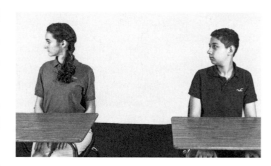

Neck Rotations

a. Inhale. Exhaling, rotate the head to look to the right. Inhale center. Exhale to the left. Inhale center. Exhale and turn to the right.

b. Keeping the head turned right, inhale and look up; exhale and look down. Repeat.

c. Inhale to the center. Exhaling, turn the head to the left.

d. Keeping the head turned to the left, inhale and look up; exhale and look down. Repeat.

e. Inhale to the center. Exhaling, lower the right ear toward the right shoulder. Slowly raise the right arm overhead. Lightly drape the hand over the left ear to deepen the stretch. Be gentle. Release. Repeat on the other side. Breathe in the pose.

f. Inhale the head to the center. Exhaling, lower the chin toward the chest. Inhale the head to the center. Exhaling, lower the chin toward the chest.

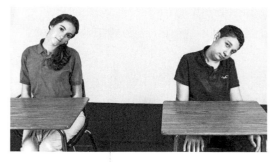

Ear to Shoulder

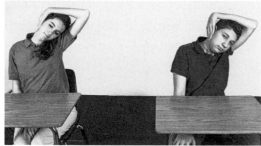

Arm over Ear

5. Spine Stretches
   - Seated Cat
     a. Angry Cat: Sit sideways in your chair with your hands on your thighs. Press into your hands and stretch your fingers like claws. Inhale. With your exhalation, tuck your chin into your throat and round your back, like an angry cat.

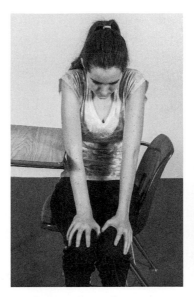 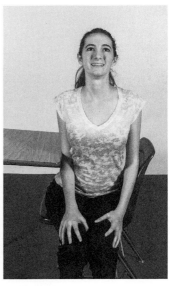

Angry Cat   Happy Cat

     b. Happy Cat: Now take a deep breath in, look up, and smile like a happy cat. (Younger children may enjoy meowing in this pose.) Repeat each pose twice more.

   - Standing Sequence
     a. Chair Shoulder Stretch: Stand with your back to your chair, holding onto it behind you. Gently walk away from your chair to open your shoulders in front.

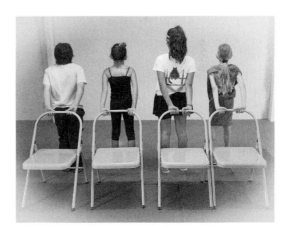

Chair Shoulder Stretch

     b. Chair Down Dog (see photo p. 193): Facing the back of your chair, drape your hands over the top. Take a few steps backward keeping your feet under your hips. Breathe and stretch your back without dropping your head. Walk forward to release the pose.

6. Yoga Singing (standing or seated): Singing these sounds has a balancing effect on the body (Paul, 2004), extends the exhalation, and opens the throat area. When teaching yoga singing, you may use visual cues, printed

in large letters on card stock, or list the sounds on the board (Goldberg, 2013). Sounds:

O (as in home)

Oo (as in too)

Ah (as in ma)

A (as in stay)

E (as in me)

M (as in yum)

N (as in sun)

a. After an inhalation, say O for the duration of the exhalation. Inhale, and exhale the sound Oo. Continue, breathing in and then repeating each sound with an exhalation, O to N.

b. After students have mastered the individual sounds, teach combinations. Practice singing O and Oo with a single exhalation. Then combine O, Oo, and Ah in one exhalation, and so forth. Adding sounds increases the duration of the exhalation, but take care not to render your students breathless.

c. When singing all the sounds together, add a circular arm sweep.

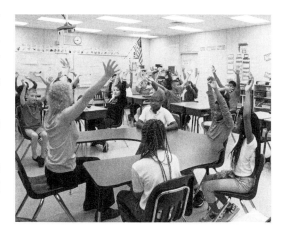

Arm Sweep

i. Begin with arms down at their sides, palms facing out for the sound O.

ii. Sweep the arms open to the sides with Oo.

iii. Continue in a large circle upward singing Ah, A, E until the arms are overhead.

iv. Singing M, N, bring the palms together in Tree Hands and lower to the center of the chest.

v. Inhaling, lower the arms to the sides and repeat.

You may sweep the arms slowly, pausing for a breath after each sound. Gradually, practice combining as many of the sounds as the students can repeat comfortably with a single exhalation.

7. High Striker (standing): This is based on a carnival attraction where contes-

tants use a mallet to strike a puck at the bottom of a scale, hoping it will reach the top for a prize (see Chapter 17).

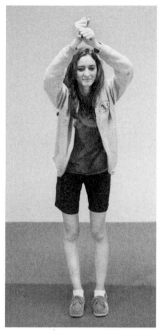

a. Bring your hands to your neck or shoulders, anywhere that you feel tension or discomfort. Breathe.

b. With your hands, collect that tension and "throw" it onto the ground.

c. Repeat once or twice, with the hands returning to the same place or to other locations (lower back, abdomen).

d. Gather up all the tension that you've thrown down, making a heap by your feet.

e. Pick up your striker (similar to a croquet mallet) and take a deep breath in.

f. Exhaling with a loud "huh" sound, slam your striker toward the ground, sending tension flying. Repeat once or twice.

g. To be sure all of the tension has been released, stomp on your pile and scatter away the last bits.

High Striker

h. Stand quietly for a moment and observe your breathing.

8. Forgiveness meditation: Letting go. When someone hurts you, it can be hard to let go of feelings of anger and frustration. Harboring resentment, however, consumes a lot of your energy. One question to consider is how

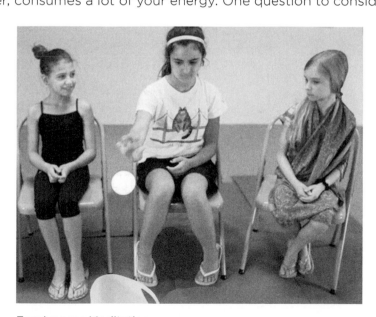

Forgiveness Meditation

much more of your emotional reserves and time is that individual worth? Might you be better served by letting those feelings go? This is not the same as forgetting. Rather, it's the process of releasing negativity associated with an event or person so that you feel better.

a. Cut paper into various sized strips.

b. On each sheet, draw a private symbol for an event that has caused you pain.

c. Crush each piece into a ball.

d. Form a circle with chairs or on the floor and place an empty wastebasket in the center.

e. One student at a time, silently throw your paper into the basket, imagining it's your anger.

f. Take a deep breath in and out after each student's turn.

9. Huh Breath three times

Fun

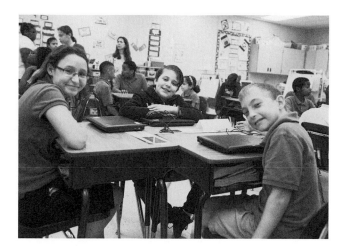

Fun

MANY OF THE usual sources of fun have been eliminated from school. Physical education, music, art, and extracurricular clubs and activities have somehow been rendered unnecessary in many school curricula. Emphasis has been shifted to grades and test scores, although these are clearly not the full measure of any child.

Stimulation and enjoyment are important ingredients in developing an environment for optimal learning. A student who is engaged is more alert and open to participation. Creating a balance between work and play also helps prevent mental fatigue and facilitates students' capacity to absorb new information. Building a sense of community within classes promotes social and emotional learning and improves behavior. Creating an atmosphere of cooperation rather than competition mitigates some of the stress inherent in scholastic settings.

Classroom yoga breaks afford opportunities to interject a few minutes of fun into a student's school day. In so doing, many teachers have found that students' attention is improved, along with conduct, academic performance, and social interaction. In taking a yoga break for students, teachers also share in the laughter and relaxation.

Practice 1: Make a Friend Laugh

When you laugh, you breathe deeply and give your body a workout. It feels good.

1. Tell a joke or funny story to a partner.
2. Write a humorous story or poem to share with your class.

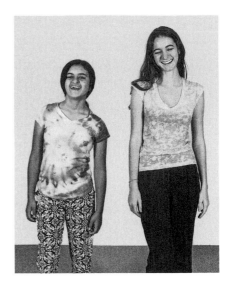

Make a Friend Laugh

Practice 2: Blowing Bubbles

When was the last time most of your students blew bubbles? In addition to having fun, this practice is useful in learning control of the breath. Each student will need a bubble ring, some bubble solution (dish soap and water), and a paper towel beneath it.

Begin with a discussion of the different ways that we breathe and how they serve us (see Unit 1).

1. How many bubbles can you send out by exhaling slowly and steadily?
2. How about with a big burst of breath?
3. Can you blow bubbles if you are out of breath?
4. Find the most efficient form of exhalation for blowing bubbles.

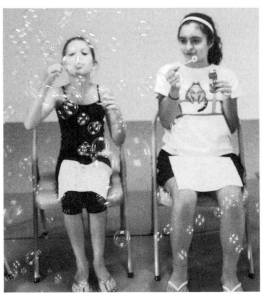

Bubbles

Practice 3: Silly Names

Each student will give himself or herself a silly name that goes along with the real name. For example, Peter could add Junkfood Eater to his name; Joel might be Jokey Joel; Mark will add Music Maker. Who can recite all the silly names of their classmates?

Fun Lessons

1. Huh Breath three times
2. Ocean Waves: Have you been to the ocean? Even on a calm day, there is continuous motion. The waves roll in and out, in a constant rhythmic fashion.
   a. Imagine that you are the ocean, and your arms are the waves.
   b. Create a rhythm, like ocean waves, with your arms and hands.
      i. First make it a rough, busy rhythm.
      ii. Begin to slow it down.
      iii. Gradually, make just the slightest motion.
   c. Create a rhythm with your own breathing like the ocean.
      i. On a rough windy day.
      ii. On a calm, peaceful day.
      iii. Imagine the sound of the waves as you breathe in and out.
3. Cooperation versus competition: Partner yoga. Select postures from this list that are appropriate for your classroom. Unless specified, these may be done with shoes on. You may want to provide students advance notice to dress for floor partner postures on a designated day.
   • Partner Standing Poses
      a. Partner Tree Supported: This is easier with partners of approximately the same height. Stand shoulder to shoulder with your partner, holding the inside hands. One partner will be the support tree,

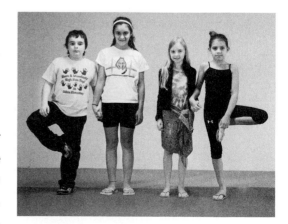

Partner Tree Supported

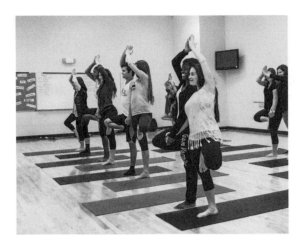

Partner Tree Balance

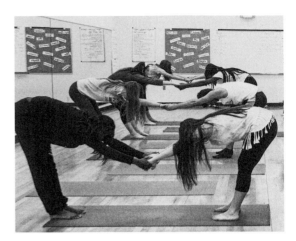

Partner Down Dog

keeping both feet on the ground. Breathe with your partner. The balance partner finds a focal point for his eyes and lifts his outside foot into low tree (at the shin or ankle) or high tree (above the knee). Use your partner for support, but find your own balance. Change roles so that each partner has a chance to balance with support.

a. Partner Tree Balance: In this variation, you start in the same way as above, but this time both partners raise their outside foot into low or high tree position. Work together and when you are ready, bring the outside hands together and elevate them. Stand and breathe. Lower and switch sides.

c. Partner Down Dog: Stand facing your partner, holding hands. Slowly begin to back away from each other, stretching your arms. Stabilize your feet under your hips as you stretch your back away from your partner. Communicate to be certain each partner is comfortable.

• Partner Seated Poses

a. Partner Balance Beam: This posture is done on hands and knees, facing your partner. Each partner rests the right hand on the partner's left shoulder for support. Raise your left leg straight behind you. Release and repeat on the other side.

b. Partner Pretzel: Begin seated on the ground, face to face. Each partner brings your right arm behind your back. With your left hand, reach

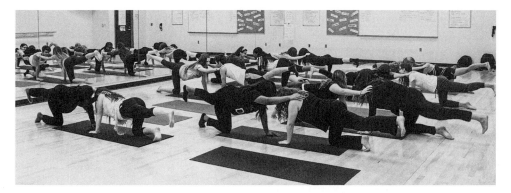

Partner Balance Beam

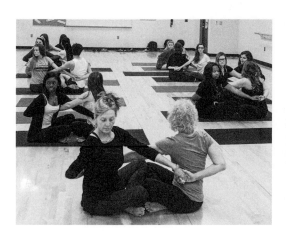

Partner Pretzel

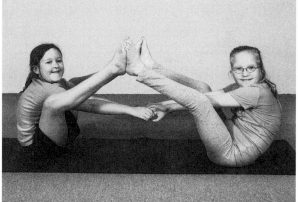

Flying Bats

across toward your partner's right hand and take hold. Ever so gently, twist your upper body to the right. Release and reverse.

c. Flying Bats: Start by sitting on the floor with shoes removed. Face your partner and hold hands inside your knees. Touch the bottom of one foot to your partner's. Slowly raise your leg up; then lower. Repeat on the other side. If this is comfortable, raise both legs. Hold on, and remember to breathe. Come down slowly and release hands.

d. Lawn Chair: This posture is done seated on the floor with your back to your partner. As one

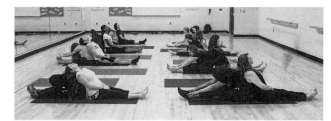

Lawn Chair

partner starts to hinge forward, the other leans back as if resting on a lawn chair. Breathe in the position and change. Take care not to push or strain in the pose. If students are more comfortable, they may bend their knees in this position.

4. Silly Moves Seated

a. Fast feet: Stretch your ankles by pointing your toes toward the floor; now toward your knees. Switch back and forth and pick up some speed. Continue with the feet moving in opposite directions. How fast can you go?

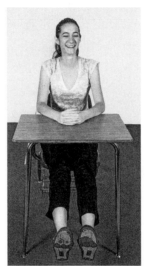

Fast Feet

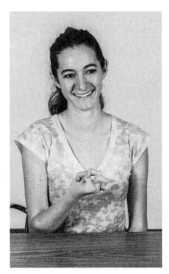

Finger Gymnastics

b. Finger gymnastics: Relax your fingers with a slight bend at the knuckles. Cross your right forefinger over your right thumb. Cross your right middle finger over your right forefinger. Now cross the ring finger over the middle. The pinkie over the ring. Avoid if there's discomfort. Release and try the other hand.

c. Palm stretch and lean: Interlace your fingers and turn the palms out. Stretch your arms overhead and float them—from side to side, side to side.

d. Butterfly hands: Imagine that your hands are like butterflies. Let them soar all around you.

e. Neck Pillow Lean: Hold onto the opposite elbow and raise your arms overhead. Let your head rest against your forearms. Ahhh. Now lean from side to side.

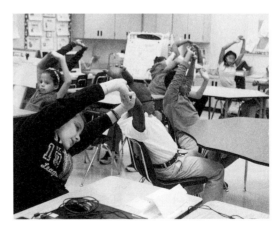

Palm Stretch and Lean

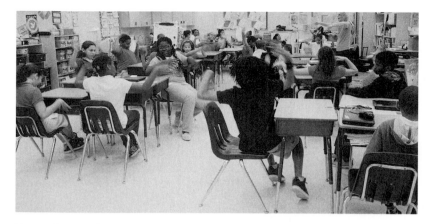

Butterfly Hands

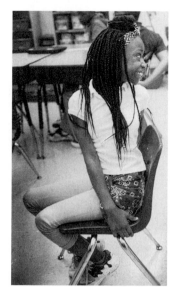

Seated Pretzel 2

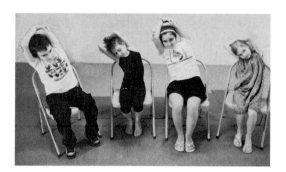

Neck Pillow Lean

f. Seated Pretzel 2: Drape your left arm over the back of your chair. Reach your right arm across your body to hold onto your chair seat. Twist your pretzel to the left. Look left: How far can you see? Now turn your head to the right, still twisting left. Once again, turn your head to the left: How far can you see? Any change? Release and reverse.

g. Open arms: Untwist and stretch your arms as wide open to the sides as you can.

h. Self-Hug: Then give yourself a hug. Release and hug with the opposite arm on top.

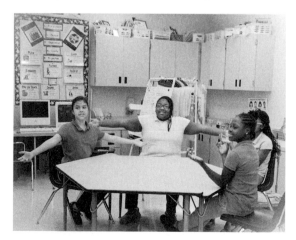

Open Arms

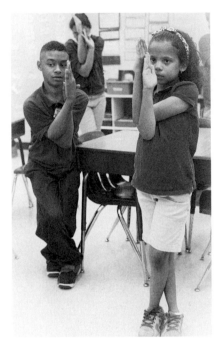
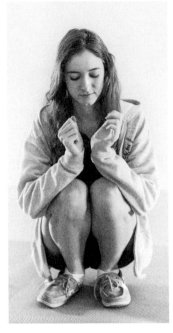
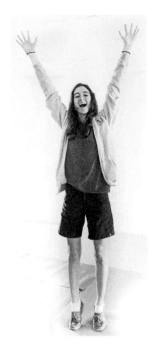

Eagle   Volcano Squat   Volcano Leap

5. Silly Moves Standing

a. Eagle: Cross your right arm over the left at the elbow. Then cross the wrists or bring the backs of the hands together. Cross your left foot over your right ankle, touching the toes to the floor. If you're feeling adventurous, bend your knees like an eagle swooping down toward its prey. Repeat on the other side.

b. Volcano Squat: Squat down like a mound of earth. Imagine that you've been here like this for a long time.

c. Volcano Leap: Start to feel a rumble inside yourself. Rumble, rumble, rumble. Begin to sway slightly from side to side with your hips and arms. Feel the heat gathering from the earth beneath you. Feel your insides bubbling up, and up, and up until they burst upward in an explosion of lava. Leap up high.

d. Fast Twister (see photo p. 215): The weather conditions are changing quickly. It's a twister! Fly your arms out as you twist from side to side.

e. Fruit Picking: If you are hungry, there's an easy solution: Pick some fruit. Reach up high for a delicious apple; out to the sides for oranges, and down low for berries. Now put all of your fruit in a pile. Stomp, stomp, stomp to make jam. Make a jam sandwich and enjoy.

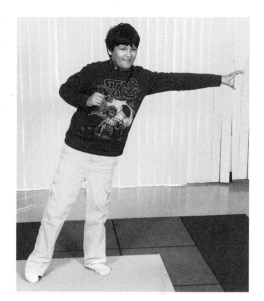

Fruit Picking

6. Shake Shake Shake (for more details, see Chapter 17.) You may do this standing or seated. Shake each area in isolation.

a. On the right side, shake the fingers, hand, wrist, elbow, upper arm, and shoulder. Shake out the entire arm. Repeat on left.

b. On the right side, shake the toes, foot, ankle, shin, knee, thigh. Shake out the entire leg. Repeat on left.

c. Shake the chin, the cheeks, the eyes, the ears, the hair, the face, and the head fully. (Take care if standing because this may affect balance.)

d. Shake the back of the body; shake the front of the body.

7. Shake it out: Now put it all together! Shake, shake, shake the whole body.

8. Make some noise (see Chapter 17 for details)

a. Quiet Hands: Begin in Tree Hands, palms together, sitting quietly. Take a deep breath.

b. Noisy Hands: Exhaling, begin to make the sound Ah. As you open your hands, get louder, louder, louder!

c. Quiet Hands: Gradually bring your palms together, getting softer, softer, softer. When your palms come together, sit quietly.

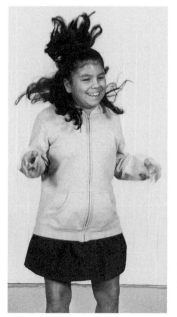

Shake It Out

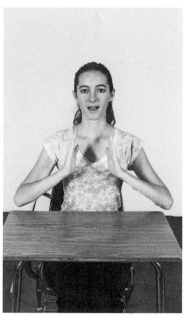

Noisy Hands

d. Close your eyes. Take soft belly breaths and listen to the quiet.

9. Smile Meditation: In *Yoga Skills for Therapists*, Amy Weintraub describes the benefit of a simple smile. The body's biochemistry is altered by facial expression, and a smile can give your "feel good hormones . . . a boost" (2012, p. 72). With permission, I have adapted Amy's technique slightly for use with children (Goldberg, 2013, p. 254). All breathing is through the nose.

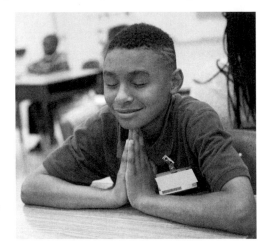

a. Breathe in; breathe out and tuck your chin way down into your chest.

b. Breathe in and out, feeling a smile start at the corners of your mouth.

c. Breathe in and lift up your chin.

Smile Meditation

d. Breathe out and show me your beautiful smile!

10. Huh Breath three times

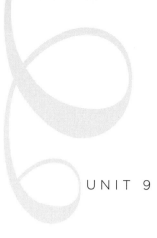

UNIT 9

Intention

THE POWER OF thought has been acknowledged throughout history. From the philosophy of ancient Rome, "Such as are your habitual thoughts, such also will be the character of your mind" (Marcus Aurelius); ancient India, "What a man thinketh, that he is" (Upanishads); the King James Bible, "For as he thinketh in his heart, so is he" (Proverbs 23:7); early modern European philosophy, "I think, therefore I am" (Descartes); American transcendentalists, "A man is what he thinks about all day long" (Ralph Waldo Emerson); modern American industrialism, "Whether you think you can or think you can't—you are right" (Henry Ford); to contemporary Zen practices, "Thoughts are the seeds of our intentions, so they are the original source of every action we perform" (Williams, 2000).

Science continues to validate the accuracy of the power of thought. In a 2005 study by Pascual-Leone, Amedi, Fregni, and Merabet, researchers discovered that mentally practicing an activity—in this case, learning to play the piano—was nearly as effective as physically performing the activity. Mental rehearsal changed subjects' brain maps and muscle memory and was especially effective when later combined with physical practice (Doidge, 2007).

As discussed earlier, research by Lazar et al. (2005), Hölzel et al. (2011), Froeliger et al. (2012), and Villemure et al. (2013) further demonstrates how malleable and responsive the brain is to yoga and mindfulness practices. How we use the mind makes a difference in how our brain works, how we feel, and how we perceive the world.

Teaching young people that they can choose the activity of their own mind is empowering. Yoga breaks are an excellent opportunity for students to set an intention—planting a thought of their choosing in their minds. In yoga, an intention is "a vow that has been birthed in the very core of your heart—the place of your deepest truth" (Silcox, 2014).

Intention and Test Anxiety

Taking or even anticipating tests can cause symptoms from knots in the stomach, muscle tension, and heart palpitations to full-blown panic attacks. Slow deep breathing and progressive muscle relaxation combined with positive imagery have long been recognized as tools to combat stress and improve focus during exams (Anxiety and Depression Association of America, 2016).

The University of Texas (UT) at Dallas Student Counseling Center (2016) suggests reducing test anxiety by learning and practicing relaxation techniques before tests. In addition, the counseling center notes the importance of monitoring negative thoughts, which provoke anxiety: "Research shows that test anxiety can be reduced if these negative thoughts can be replaced by constructive thoughts" (UT Dallas Counseling Center, 2016).

Combining focused movement, relaxation, and breathing exercises with intention-setting gives students increased tools to ease anxiety before or during high pressure situations throughout their day. Begin each of the following practices with a quiet moment to set an intention—something simple, positive, and supportive to the student's well-being. Remind them that there is power in this process.

Practice 1: Intention Journal

For one week, begin each day with an intention—a positive thought that pertains just to you. For example, "I will smile often today"; "I acknowledge my fears and my strengths"; "I tune in to my inner quiet." Keep a journal describing this practice and how it makes you feel.

Practice 2: Research on Thinking

Research (a) the power of thinking and/or (b) how meditation and yoga change the brain. See the references above for specific studies or philosophers to explore. Refer to Part III in this book. (This may be a written assignment or oral presentation.)

Practice 3: The Power of Mental Rehearsal

Construct an experiment in your classroom inspired by the work of Pascual-Leone. Select two groups of students who have no experience with a skill such as knitting or stringing a kite. Prepare clear, step-by-step instructions on how to perform the task.

  a. Assign a physical group to review the instructions and practice performing the task for a set amount of time.
  b. Assign a mental group to review the instructions and practice performing it in their minds for a comparable amount of time.
  c. After the period of practice, ask each group to perform the task physically.
  d. Compare the results of the groups.

Intention Lessons

1. Huh Breath three times
2. Centering Breath: Use soft belly breathing as you repeat these words silently:
   a. Inhale: "calm in"; exhale: "tension out."
   b. Repeat five times.
3. Intentional Sounds (seated or standing): Singing or chanting sounds is a tool to extend the exhalation, which has a calming effect. Use these sounds to plant an intention within body and mind.
   a. Steadying: Oh
   b. Turning inward: Hum

     c. Overcoming challenge: Yay

     d. Soothing: Ah

     e. Energizing: Ee

     f. Acceptance: Ooh

4. Finger Press: Combining physical touch with a mental intention intensifies its effectiveness. Select a simple, positive word or phrase for this exercise. Silently repeat your positive statement as you press your right thumb to your right forefinger. Silently repeat as you continue to press your thumb to each of the fingers on your right hand. Continue, using the left hand, until you have set this intention eight times.

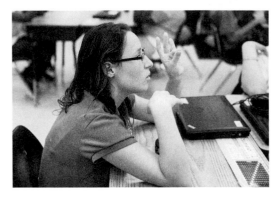

Finger Press

Creative Relaxation: Easing Test Anxiety

Adapted with permission from *Yoga Therapy for Children with Autism and Special Needs* (Goldberg, 2013, pp. 213–215), these routines have been implemented successfully with students in upper elementary grades through college. See Chapter 16 for additional information about mental rehearsal before tests.

5. Before test: Mental rehearsal. Make a simple affirmation before the test such as "I will do my best"; "I am focused"; "I am prepared."

     a. Mentally suggest that you are calm and relaxed; you are prepared to do well.

     b. Grounding check: Sit with your feet firmly on the floor and your body fully supported in the chair.

     c. Posture check: 90-degree angles at your hips and knees; sit upright with an open chest.

     d. Breathing check: Use soft belly breathing through the nostrils to stay alert and relaxed.

6. During test: Calming tools. If your mind starts to wander or you feel anxious, do one of these quick stress relievers for a count of 3 seconds or less.

Remain quiet, without disturbing your neighbor, with just the slightest movement. Then return immediately to your work.

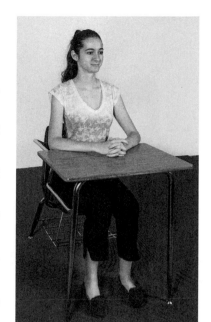

a. Grounded sitting: Check your posture—feet on floor, back straight, belly relaxed.

b. Yawn: Stretch your face with a deep breath in; sigh it out.

c. Shoulder circles: Circle once in each direction without hands.

d. Breathing check: Am I breathing? Take one or two soft belly breaths.

e. Finger release: Wiggle and stretch the fingers, keeping the hands in your lap.

f. Open chest: Take a deep breath as you lean into the back of the chair—no arms for this one.

g. Feet release: Wiggle your toes.

Grounded Sitting

7. Between tests: Seated

a. Neck stretches (see photo p. 222): Turn to look over your right shoulder. Inhale and look up; exhale and look down. Repeat. Inhale to the center; exhale and look left. Inhale and look up; exhale and look down. Repeat.

b. Elbow pumping (see photo p. 176): Bring the hands onto the shoulders. Inhaling, open the elbows; exhaling, close. Then circle the elbows and reverse.

c. Finger pull: Give your fingers a gentle stretch by pulling each one.

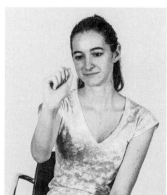

d. Wrist circles: Making a loose fist, rotate the wrist in each direction. Then circle with a relaxed hand. Repeat with the other wrist.

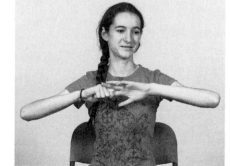

e. Palm Stretch and Lean (see photo p. 232): Interlace the fingers and stretch the palms

Finger Pull

away from you. Then stretch the arms overhead and sway them from side to side.

Wrist Circles

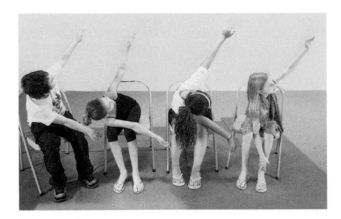

Seated Windmill

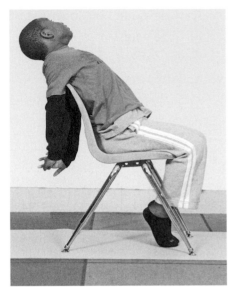

Chair Half Fish

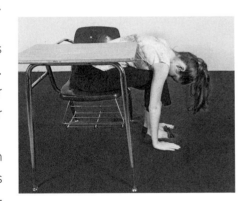

Folded Leaf

f. Seated Windmill: Reach your right hand across your body past your left knee or toward your left shin. Raise your left arm up toward the ceiling. Lower and repeat on the other side.

g. Chair Half Fish: Clasp your hands behind your back and open your chest. If this is not comfortable, hang your arms out to the sides and press your back against your chair.

h. Chair Folded Leaf: Turn sideways in your chair and gently walk your hands down your legs until you are comfortable.

i. Feet release

  i. Point the toes toward your nose, then toward the floor. Repeat.

  ii. Circle your ankles in one direction; reverse.

  iii. Wiggle your toes and shake out your feet.

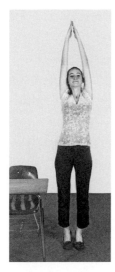

Stretch Tall

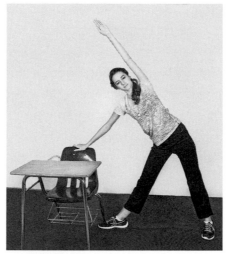

Desk Triangle

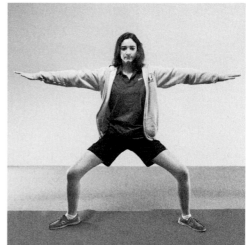

Five-Pointed Star

8. Between tests: Standing

   a. Stretch tall: Reach your arms up high, palms together.

   b. Yawn: Yawn and stretch your face. Take another deep breath in and out.

   c. Desk Triangle: Stand to the left side of your desk, touching your chair with your right hand. Widen your legs and point your toes to the right. Elevate your left arm alongside your ear. Exhaling, lean gently to the right, keeping both sides of your body long. Inhale upright. Release. Switch sides.

   d. Wide Stance: Stand with your feet wide apart and stretch your arms out to the sides.

   e. Five-Pointed Star: From Wide Stance, with your toes pointing outward, inhale. Exhale, and bend your knees out to the sides, unless there's discomfort. Inhale and straighten; exhale and bend. Repeat once more.

   f. Tall Tree: Start in stretch tall position, with your palms together; arms overhead. Breathe in the pose: Inhale up on the toes; exhale and lower the heels. Keeping the arms up, repeat the heel lift for up to three breaths. Then, with an exhalation, lower the heels and the hands.

   g. Chair Down Dog (see photo p. 193): Hold onto the back of your chair and walk your feet away, stretching your arms and back. Keep your head between your hands.

h. Chair Windmill (see photo p. 207): From Chair Down Dog, lower your right hand to your left shin. Come back into Chair Down Dog; repeat with the left hand.

i. Chair Up Dog (see photo p. 214): , Standing about a shin length away, hold on to the back of your chair with both hands. Take a deep breath in, drawing your shoulder blades together and opening your chest. Look upward, but don't let your head hang back. Take another breath in the pose and release with the exhalation.

j. Bellows Breath (see photos p. 180): Interlace your hands behind your head. Inhale and look up. Exhale and look down. Repeat.

k. Twister (see photo p. 215): Let your arms fly as you swing from side to side.

9. After the test: What's done is done.

a. Run in place. Work up a sweat.

b. Shake it out: Let everything go!

c. Visualize the best outcome.

d. Whenever you think about the test, take a Huh Breath. Remind yourself that you have done all you can for now.

10. Huh Breath three times

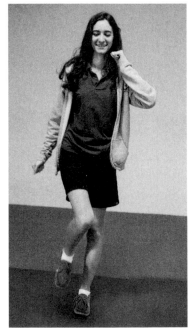

Run In Place

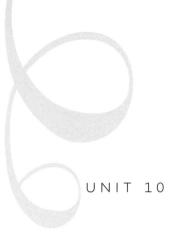

UNIT 10

Reset

HAVE YOU EVER sat in front of the television channel surfing, mindlessly switching from show to show every few minutes? That's how a lot of us spend our inner time, too—shifting from thought to thought, mindlessly, without even knowing it.

Pushing the reset button on your phone or computer clears its contents and opens a clean page. You can learn to do something similar through yoga. Breathing exercises help clear negative thoughts. Energizing postures can get you out of a slump, and calming poses are useful for shifting your body and mind to a more peaceful setting. Yoga and mindfulness practices such as breathing, posture, relaxation, and meditation have been shown to reduce rumination and anxiety among youth (Mendelson et al., 2010).

Meditation is an important technique for controlling the activity of the mind. It takes many forms, including movement, music, breath awareness, and quiet sitting. A commonly used tool in meditation is a mantra—the repetition of a word or phrase of your own choosing. According to psychologist Lawrence LeShan (1974) in his book *How to Meditate*, repeating a mantra keeps the mind focused on one thing at a time; this is one-pointedness.

Originating from the Sanskrit word for mind, the term "mantra" has entered today's lexicon. Merriam-Webster defines it as a word or phrase used to express a personal or professional motto. A classic mantra within children's literature is the refrain from *The Little Engine That Could*: "I think I can, I think I can" (Piper, 1976). Repeating this positive thought encouraged the little engine to attempt and achieve a difficult feat.

What's Your Mantra?

Most of us have more than one mantra, a word or phrase, rolling around inside our heads. Unfortunately, these thoughts are not always positive.

Let me give you a personal example. Punctuality is often a challenge for me. Racing against the clock, I usually hear these words in my mind: "I'm going to be late; I'm going to be late." This recurring thought makes me feel even more stressed as I rush to get ready or weave my car through heavy traffic.

One day it occurred to me that by repeating this phrase, I was actually affirming a negative pattern that I did not want to reinforce. So I changed my mantra. Whenever I heard the refrain "I'm going to be late" start up in my mind, I consciously changed it to "I will arrive safely on time." Resetting my inner thinking has made a difference. While I still have a challenging relationship with time, this altered phrase helps me drive more carefully and arrive in a much less anxious state.

Many people, especially adolescents, are plagued with self-doubt and criticism. Their ruminations sound more like this: "I'm not good enough." "That's too hard for me." "This is never going to work." Most individuals don't recognize the frequency or power of these internal refrains.

Do you have a word or phrase rolling through your mind that is not useful? If you catch yourself thinking, "I'll never be able to do that," you might reset that thought to "I'd like to try" or "I accept that challenge." Those words alone will not ensure your getting something difficult accomplished, but they may help you, as they did me, reframe your outlook from negative to positive and reduce rather than intensify your levels of stress.

Remember, no word or phrase will replace the effort required to bring about your desired outcome. But you can reset the language you use to describe the process. Observe what is happening inside your own head and reframe negative or intrusive thoughts; choose words that support you.

Practice 1: Discussion—What Is Your Mantra?

Do you have a thought or phrase that encourages you? Do you have others that do not serve you?

Practice 2: Reframing Journal

Experiment with resetting your internal channel from "I can't" to "I'd like to"; from "this will never" to "this could"; from "I'm not" to "I am." Keep a journal for a week, recording each time you hear an unproductive thought in your head. Reframe that thought to something useful and positive. Write it down and repeat it silently. See if it changes how you feel. If it's helpful, use it; if not, try something else.

Reset Lessons

1. Huh Breath three times
2. Follow the breath: In this calming sequence, hold each hand position for three breaths.
   a. Place your hands on your belly, one atop the other. Notice if or how the hands move with the breath.
   b. Rest your hands on your lower ribs at the sides, with your fingers pointed forward and your thumbs back. Inhale and exhale, feeling the movement in your hands.

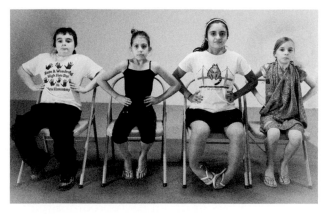

Lower Ribs

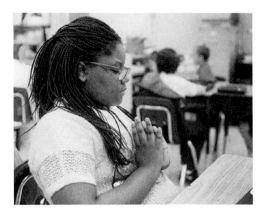

Sternum

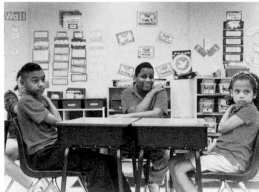

Shoulder

c. Place the palms together in the center of the chest, thumbs at the sternum with the fingers pointing upward. Inhale and exhale, feeling the movement in your chest.

d. Rest your right palm over the top of your left shoulder, with your fingers pointing down toward your shoulder blades. Inhale and exhale, feeling the movement in your hand and shoulder. Switch sides.

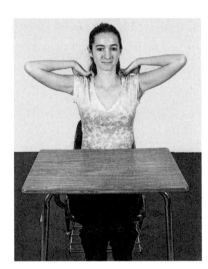

Elbow Lift

e. Drape your fingers over your shoulders with the elbows lifted out to the sides. Inhale and exhale, feeling the movement in your hands and shoulders.

f. Bring your hands back to your belly. Inhale and exhale, feeling the movement in your hands.

3. Take 5 (from *S.T.O.P. and Relax*, with permission, Goldberg et al., 2006): When you feel your emotions churning out of control, stop and take five slow, deep breaths. Use your fingers to count each breath. Breathe in and out silently through your nostrils. Repeat as needed.

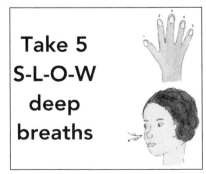

Take 5 S-L-O-W deep breaths

"Take 5" S.T.O.P. and Relax

4. Yoga breaks for transitions: Change, whether unexpected or predictable, can be disturbing, especially for students with anxiety or exceptional needs. Yoga breaks may help ease their transition from one activity to another. Energizing postures help increase alertness before an exam. Calming postures are useful before settling down to work. Breathing exercises help many students regain their focus.

    Yoga breaks can also be used as stress reliever in between demanding activities for students of all abilities. The following are examples of "unwasting time," as discussed in Chapter 16.

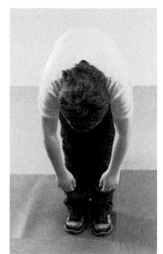

Rag Doll

  a. At the beginning of class: Rag Doll before sitting. Let your arms and head hang down toward the ground, unless inversions are contraindicated.

  b. Refocusing attention: Follow your thumb (see photo p. 210). Follow your thumb with your eyes as you slowly stretch your arm out to your right side; then left. Keep your focus on your thumb as you move it in a slow circle clockwise; then counterclockwise. Repeat with other thumb.

  c. After testing: Silent Lion (see p. 221). With an inhalation, squeeze your eyes, your mouth and lips tightly closed. Exhaling, stretch your mouth and eyes open wide.

  d. At the end of class: Seated Pretzel 2 before getting up. Twist in each direction in your seat (see photo p. 233).

  e. While the class is waiting in line: Tree Breathing (see pp. 176–77). Bring the palms together. Inhale, elevate the hands; exhale lower. Repeat.

  f. Unexpected schedule change: three Huh Breaths before new activity. Inhale and elevate the shoulders; exhale and drop with a "huh."

  g. After gym class or assembly: Folded Leaf in seat (see photo p. 242). Sit sideways in your chair. Walk your hands down toward the floor.

  h. Before lunch: Umbrella Squeeze or Half Fish. Standing, clasp your hands behind your back, take a deep breath, and open your chest in Umbrella Squeeze (see photo p. 184). Seated, lean back and clasp your hands behind the chair in Half Fish (see photo p. 182), or let them hang over the back of the seat. Take a deep breath in and out.

  i. After lunch: Bellows Breath 2 (see photo p. 180). Chin tuck: Interlace your fingers and clasp your hands behind your head. Inhale in position. With an exhalation, tuck your chin down toward your throat. Breathe gently in the pose.

j. Midclass Wake-Up Break: Palm Stretch and Lean (see photo p. 181). Seated or standing, interlace your fingers and turn your palms out. Stretch your arms overhead with an inhalation; lean left with an exhalation. Repeat, leaning from side to side.

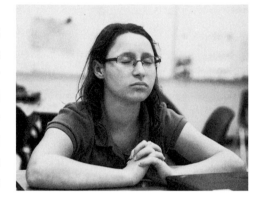

k. Before writing assignments: Soft belly breathing. Find a comfortable position in your chair. Close your eyes and focus on the quiet sound of the breath as it enters your body through your nostrils, softly filling your belly. As you exhale, feel the breath leave through your nostrils as your belly gets smaller. Repeat twice more.

Before Writing

5. Reset: Calming Sequence seated

   a. Huh Breath three times

   b. Parachute Breath slow: Start with the arms relaxed at your sides. Inhale, turn the palms out and sweep the arms up alongside you and overhead, palms touching. Exhaling, turn the palms out and float the arms back to your sides. Repeat three to five times.

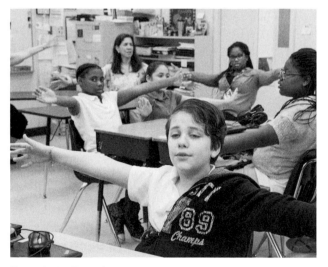

Parachute Breath

   c. Butterfly Hands: Let your hands float all around you like butterflies.

d. Butterfly Meditation: Sit very quietly with your hands resting on your desk, palms up. Imagine that you are sitting in a beautiful garden, surrounded by butterflies. If you sit very still, a butterfly will land right in the palm of each hand. Gaze at the butterfly in your right hand. Lift it toward you, moving slowly so as not to disturb the butterfly. Lower it back down. Now, gaze at the beautiful butterfly resting in the palm of your left hand. Lift it slowly, noticing the colors and shapes of your resting butterfly. Lower it back down. Repeat twice more. Now, very gently, blow into each hand so that your butterflies fly off to visit the flowers in the garden.

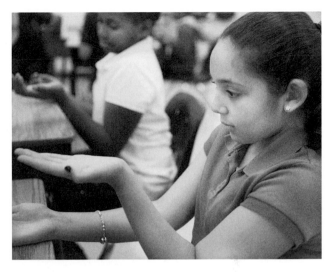

Butterfly Meditation

e. Arm stretch: Reach both arms up high and take a deep inhalation.

f. Half Moon Wrist: Grasp your right wrist with your left hand. Inhale in position; exhale and lean to the left. Inhale upright. Change hands and lean to the right. Repeat on each side.

g. Half Fish Open Arms (see photo p. 216): Let your arms dangle behind you as you lean back in your chair; breathe deeply.

h. Bellows Breath 2: Chin tuck (see photo p. 180). Inhale as you interlace your hands behind your head. Exhaling, tuck your chin into your chest. Take three soft belly breaths in this position. Inhaling, release the hands and let your head float to a neutral position.

6. Reset: Energizing sequence standing
   a. Huh Breath three times

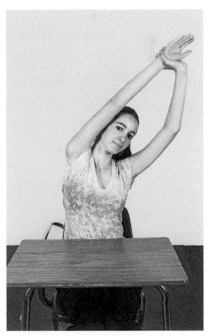

Half Moon Wrist

b. Crane: Stand on both feet and find a focal point for your eyes. Shift the weight to your right foot and elevate your left foot slightly off the ground. Relax your wrists. Lower your left foot and lift your right. Keep your focus. Shift from foot to foot as slowly or quickly as you can do comfortably. Remember to breathe.

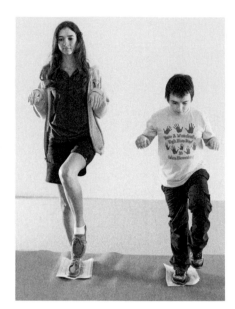

Crane

c. Dancer (see photo p. 209): Standing with your left hip alongside your desk, place your left hand on your desk or chair. Stand up straight and take a deep breath. Exhaling, bend your right knee and grasp your foot or ankle with your right hand. Inhale and exhale in the pose. Release, turn around, and repeat on the other side.

d. Twister Fast: Let your arms fly to the sides as you twist fast. Now slow it down.

e. Windmill: Stand with your feet wide apart, arms open wide. As you lower your right hand toward your left thigh or shin, stretch your left arm up high. Reverse. Repeat twice on each side.

f. Bellows Breath 1: Head rest standing (see photo p. 183): Interlace your hands behind your head. Inhale and look up. Hold the pose. Breathe in and out.

g. Shake it out: Shake out your whole body.

7. Breathing four count: Keeping your mind focused on your breathing takes a great deal of concentration. Sit comfortably, taking soft belly breaths. For this practice, repeat the word "and" silently each time you inhale. Count each exhalation silently, starting with

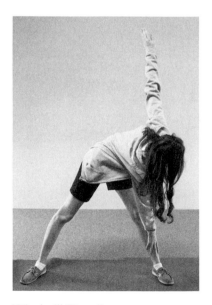

Windmill Standing

one. When you reach four, start again at one. Count to yourself as you listen to these instructions:

a. Inhale "and"; exhale, "1."

b. Inhale "and"; exhale, "2."

c. Inhale "and"; exhale, "3."

d. Inhale "and"; exhale, "4."

e. Inhale "and"; exhale, "1."

Continue silently until you hear the signal to stop. If you lose your count anywhere along the way, start again with 1.

8. Thought Balloons: Use soft belly breathing while sitting upright comfortably.

a. Observe your inhalation and exhalation.

b. Notice if a distracting thought creeps into your mind.

c. Without judgment, acknowledge the thought.

d. In your imagination, place the thought in a big colorful balloon and watch it float out of your mind.

e. Return your attention to soft belly breathing.

f. Release thoughts as they come into your mind in balloons of all colors and sizes.

9. Huh Breath three times

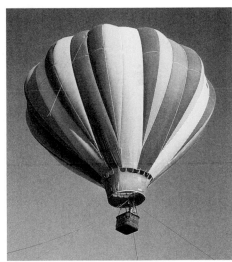

Thought Balloon

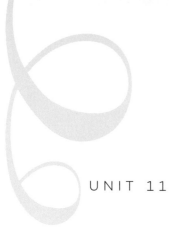

UNIT 11

Sense of Self

I N YOGA, THERE is a great deal of emphasis on authenticity. After kindness, the second of the Guidelines for Classroom Yoga Breaks (Chapter 14) is "be truthful." The example of Gandhi is that of the compassionate warrior—one who fiercely adhered to his personal creed of nonviolence and truthfulness.

Throughout this curriculum, we encourage students to discover and pursue their personal path. Developing their own sense of self is more important than succeeding by following someone else's.

This struggle for personal identity is the work of adolescence. Sometimes teens vacillate between apathy and intense involvement. They may throw themselves headfirst into one activity to the exclusion of their schoolwork, drop everyone else for a girlfriend or boyfriend, or abruptly switch between different groups of friends. Their personal values may appear to shift depending upon which group they associate with. It can be difficult for teens to find the balance in their connections with others while still maintaining a sense of themselves.

It's not uncommon for young people to become so focused on what others are thinking and saying that they disregard their own needs and values. This sometimes puts them at risk. Through self-awareness practices, teens can learn to be attentive to the feelings and needs of others without losing—or harming—themselves in the process.

Establishing Emotional Boundaries

Let there be spaces in your togetherness. (Gibran, 1998, p. 23)

The role of the lungs in respiration is an excellent instructional tool for teaching students about establishing emotional boundaries. As you sit breathing quietly, imagine your lungs nearly filling with each inhalation. Imagine them partially emptying with each exhalation. The lungs never completely empty, no matter how deeply we exhale. The air held in each lung after exhalation helps it retain its shape and prevents collapse.

If we apply the metaphor of the lungs to our own lives, there's a powerful message: Never empty yourself so completely that you risk collapse. If you give away too much of your time, your energy, your passion, you risk diminishing your personal reserves. Overinvolvement in another's drama could cost you your independence. Retaining your sense of self, your personal identity, is essential to navigating a balanced, healthy life.

When I took junior life saving training at summer camp, I learned how frequently a well-intended rescue attempt turns into a double drowning. We were drilled on the importance of throwing a life preserver rather than jumping into an already turbulent situation. It's always more prudent, we were instructed, to act from solid ground.

Body Image

Adolescence is a period of extraordinary physical growth. Young people find themselves inhabiting a body that is unfamiliar. Because of the rapid shifts they endure, establishing a clear identity can be especially challenging. Here again, influences from media and peers often exert pressure to conform to a physical standard that is not suitable for them.

Learning to connect to and accept one's body can be healing in many ways. In Chapter 12, we noted the role of yoga in helping students with eating disorder behaviors to become less critical of their bodies and to embrace techniques to improve their overall wellness (Cook-Cottone, 2016). We've also heard from a number of students who have improved their physical and emotional self-image after implementing yoga techniques. Strategies that promote self-acceptance also lead to greater empathy for others. This is a crucial step toward building a community of compassionate, responsible citizens.

Practice 1: Personal Support Journal

What kinds of activities make you feel better about yourself? Are these practices that enhance your well-being? Describe three things that you can do that make you feel better about yourself and support your physical and emotional health.

Commit to practicing at least one of these things daily for one week. Record the results.

Practice 2: Balanced Support

Discuss these concepts: Who fills you up and who drags you down? Are there people in your life who support you and are there for you? Are there others who take advantage of you or use up a lot of your energy? Do you have friends who sometimes lean on you and sometimes let you lean on them? Describe the balance in the relationships that are important to you. Compare that to relationships that are imbalanced.

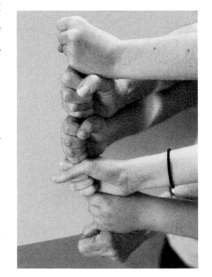

Practice 3: Feeling Stuck

1. Form circles of four to six students.
2. Every student makes a fist with both hands.
3. Taking turns, they stack their fists firmly on top of each other's fists, with thumbs upward.
4. Try to move one from the middle of the stack.

Discuss what happens.

Hand Stack

Do you ever feel stuck or weighed down by others? Consider a quotation from Kahlil Gibran: "Let there be spaces in your togetherness." What might that feel like? How can you practice this in your social interactions?

Sense of Self Lessons

1. Huh Breath three times
2. Power Breath: With a silent inhalation through the nose, imagine the breath traveling up through
   a. The soles of the feet
   b. The legs
   c. The torso
   d. The face
   e. To the top of the head
   Exhaling with a long ah sound, imagine the breath
   f. Moving out like electrical sparks
   g. Energizing your whole body
3. Personal centering: Choose a positive descriptive word that you would like to plant deep within.
   a. Inhale and silently say, "I am."
   b. Exhale and silently say your word (peace, love, kindness, strength, etc.)
   c. Repeat five times silently.
   d. Then repeat aloud three times.
4. Group balance poses: Boundaries and physical support. When you work as a team, you can often accomplish things beyond your expectations. Providing support and respecting boundaries requires a delicate balance among all participants.
   a. Shoulder-to-shoulder stance: Stand in a row with a group of classmates, shoulder to shoulder. Squeeze in close. Do you feel crowded? Supported?

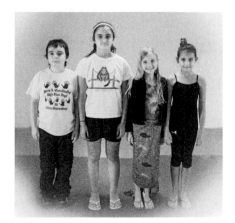

Shoulder to Shoulder

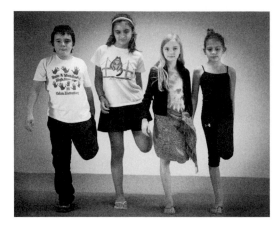

Group Dancer

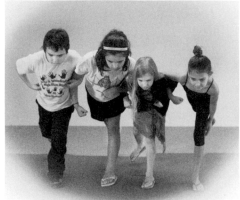

Group Warrior Balance

b. Group Dancer: Line up shoulder to shoulder alongside your classmates. Stand up straight and take a deep breath. Exhaling, bend your right knee and grasp your foot or ankle with your right hand behind your back. Inhale and exhale in the pose. Release and repeat on the other side. Try the posture on your own to compare. In what ways was it easier to do this in a group? In what ways more difficult?

c. Group Warrior 3 Balance: Stand in a row alongside your classmates. Hook arms at the elbow. Inhale in position and fix your gaze on a spot on the floor about your height in front of you. As you exhale, hinge forward on your right hip and begin to lift the left leg off the floor behind you. Breathe together. What happens if your partners let go? Repeat on the other side.

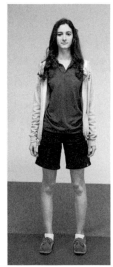

5. How do you present yourself? Consider the messages below as you practice these poses. You may substitute a personal statement that is more reflective of your sense of self in these postures.

• Mountain Stance

a. Mountain: Stand upright with your arms by your sides, your feet planted firmly on the ground beneath your hips. This sends the message, "I am strong and confident."

Mountain Stance

b. Slumped: Allow your shoulders to slump, your chest to cave, and your head to hang. This sends the message, "I can't stand up for myself."

• Focus

a. Fast Twister (see photo p. 215): Let your arms fly as you twist from side to side. This sends the message, "I'm a free spirit" or "I release that which does not serve me."

b. Tree: Use your eyes to focus on a point on the ground about the same distance as your height in front of you. Bring your weight

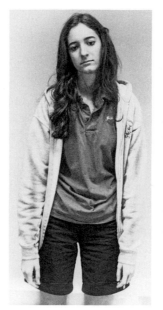 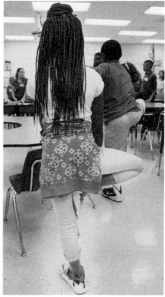

Slumped Stance   High Tree

onto your left foot. Lift your right foot and place it inside your left shin for Low Tree or inside your thigh for High Tree (not on the knee). Bring your palms together at your heart. Lower the foot and repeat on the other side. This sends the message, "I am focused and steady."

• Warrior

a. Warrior 1 back bend: Step one foot in front of the other in Warrior 1. Clasp your hands or wrists behind your back. Take your gaze toward the ceiling and lift your chest, without dropping your head back. Repeat on the other side. This sends the message, "I use my strength to bend over backward for what I care about."

b. Compassionate Warrior 2: Stand with your feet wide apart and your arms open to your sides. Turn both feet to the right. Bend

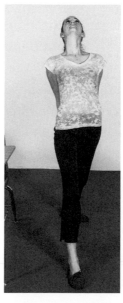 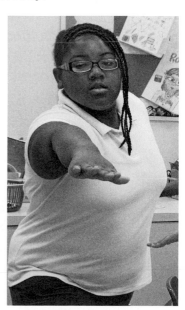

Warrior 1 Back Bend   Compassionate Warrior 2

your right knee and turn your head to look past your right hand. Feel your strength. Repeat on the left. This sends the message, "I calmly stand my ground, while aware of everything and everyone around me."

- Strength and flexibility
  a. Chair (see photo p. 192): Stand with your feet hip distance apart, hands on your knees. Bend your knees and raise your arms up alongside your ear. This sends the message, "I am strong and stable."
  b. Rag Doll (see photo p. 194): Being certain that you have space for your head, relax your arms and soften your knees. Let your upper body hang gently forward toward the ground. This sends the message, "I can let anything roll off my back."

6. Stretch Yourself

a. Arm stretch: Stretch your arms out wide to the sides.

b. Folded Leaf Open Heart: Clasp your hands behind your back and fold forward. If this is not comfortable for you, hold your wrists or forearms as you fold, or release your arms.

c. One-arm seated twist: Rest your left forearm on your desk. Elevate your right arm alongside your ear. Inhale in position. With an exhalation, slowly twist to the right. Breathe in the posture. With your next exhalation, return to center. Switch sides.

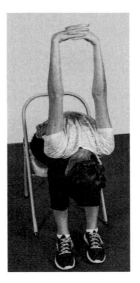
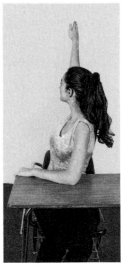

Folded Leaf Open Heart

One-Arm Seated Twist

d. Half Chair Eagle (see photo p. 201): Seated in your chair, cross your right arm over your left at the elbow. Then bend your elbows and bring the backs of the hands toward one another. Keep them in this position or cross again at the wrists and bring your palms toward one another.

e. Full Chair Eagle: Sit sideways in your chair with your arms in Half Eagle, right arm on top, Now cross your left thigh over your right. Stay in this

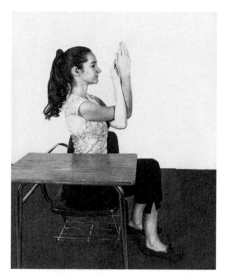

Full Chair Eagle

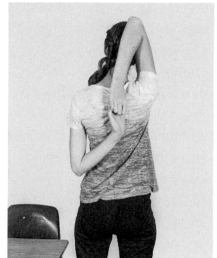

Full Cow's Head

position, or see if you can tuck your left ankle behind your right calf for a double cross. Uncross and repeat d and e on the opposite side.

f. Full Cow's Head: Raise your right arm overhead. Bend the elbow and bring your palm onto your back, reaching down your spine. Now bring the left arm behind you and bend the elbow with the back of the hand resting on your back and fingertips reaching up toward your other hand. Don't force it if you can't touch your fingers—this is a challenge. Release and reverse.

g. Half Moon One Arm, standing (see photo p. 177): Raise your right arm overhead with an inhalation. Exhaling, lean left. Inhale center and change arms. Lean to the right.

7. Peace Comes From Me Meditation, 5 minutes. This exercise is adapted from a Kundalini yoga meditation technique (Khalsa, 1996, pp. 208–209) and a self-hypnosis practice I learned from Faye Lubline in 1988. Teacher serves as time keeper in this exercise.

a. Sit with your body upright and comfortable. First try the finger presses on each hand separately. Then continue using both hands simultaneously.

b. Speaking aloud

i. Lightly touch your thumb to your first finger on both hands simultaneously and say "peace."

ii. Lightly touch your thumb and middle finger on both hands and say "comes."

iii. Lightly touch your thumb and ring finger on both hands and say "from."

iv. Lightly touch your thumb and pinky finger on both hands and say "me."

Repeat this statement with the light finger presses for 1 minute.

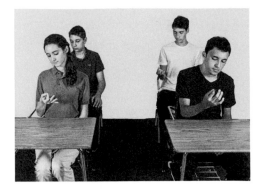

Peace Comes from Me

c. Whispering: Continue in the same manner, but this time whisper the words "Peace comes from me" for 1 minute.

d. Silence: Pressing the fingers, this time say the words silently in your own mind for 1 minute.

e. Whisper: Then whisper again for 1 minute.

f. Speak: Then speak aloud again for 1 minute.

g. Relax your hands and take three soft belly breaths. Repeat silently, "Peace comes from me" with each breath.

To abbreviate this routine, you may shorten the time to 30 seconds for each portion. For a 1-minute routine, use the finger presses and reduce the sequence to (a) whispering, (b) silence, and (c) whispering for 20 seconds each.

8. Huh Breath three times

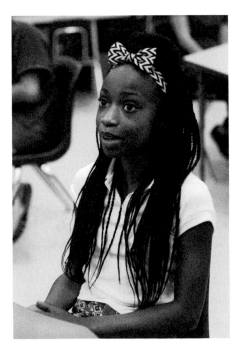

Sense of Self

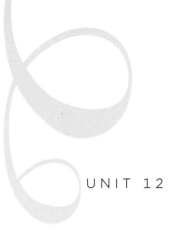

UNIT 12

In Touch

The Language of Touch

Our first language is touch. The need to be comforted, rocked, and held is as great as the need for physical nourishment for humans. When we touch or are touched by others, a feel-good hormone called oxytocin is released. Mammals deprived of touch withdraw and do not thrive. Touch is a powerful indicator of our connection with others, our sense of community. It can be used to heal or to harm.

Despite the importance of this modality, our culture limits opportunities to use touch for communication and administering comfort. In fact, much of the emphasis on touch is fear based for children: "Don't let anyone get too close. Keep your distance. Don't touch anything. Keep your hands off." Although this is often good advice, it also contributes to fear and confusion about touch.

Responsiveness to touch is an important diagnostic tool for determining certain conditions such as autism and sensory processing disorders. As discussed in Chapter 8, Temple Grandin is an individual on the autism spectrum who experienced extreme discomfort with being touched. It wasn't until she had felt the calming effects of touch herself that she learned how to comfort others. She believes that becoming more empathetic is a corollary to learning how to touch (Grandin, 2006).

How can young people learn to use this most intuitive, basic form of expression for comfort and reassurance? Permission to touch is rarely granted in school or therapeutic settings. Even in the medical profession, there is often little direct physical contact. With so much emphasis on its inappropriateness, we have become a society that is reluctant to touch.

By not teaching children about touch, we miss an important opportunity in social-emotional education. Learning to establish physical boundaries and to respect those of others could potentially mitigate episodes of bullying and other aggressive behaviors. Students need to practice and communicate about how it feels when someone is too close, how it feels to sense someone's fear of their touch, and what they might do to change either of those situations. These conversations and skills can be incorporated into classroom curricula with yoga breaks. Teaching students how to accept or refuse touch helps them establish ownership over their bodies.

Pain as Teacher

One of the biggest incentives to tuning out feelings is to avoid pain. Although living a pain-free life may sound idyllic, it is fraught with countless perils. Congenital insensitivity is a very rare genetic condition that renders individuals incapable of feeling pain. One young child with this condition was badly burned without even noticing and knocked out her own teeth by running into walls (Tresniowski, 2005).

Clearly, this is a rare case. Nevertheless, we live in a culture that encourages dismissing pain. By taking a pill or toughing it out, we are trained to ignore important information from within. Pain is, in fact, a guide, alerting us to danger and setting safe limits.

Yoga is a tool that helps young people recognize messages from within their own nervous systems. Getting in touch with themselves, they learn to distinguish between a stretch, which is a comfortable challenge, and strain, a potential source of injury. They learn to find freedom within the limitations of complex twisted postures and demanding holds. They learn to recognize and release unneeded tension from their muscles, to listen to and regulate their breathing, to find comfort within their own skin.

Practice 1: Language of Touch Discussion

Have you been touched by a poignant story? Have you ever felt that your parents were out of touch with what's important to you? Do you get touchy when people tease you? Do your friends ask you to keep in touch? Can you think of other phrases such as "soft touch" or "easy touch"? What do these mean to you?

Practice 2: Touch Can Heal or Harm

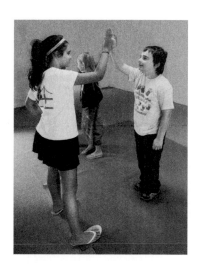

When you touch others, what message do you convey?

1. Walk around the room and exchange handshakes. What do others observe through your touch?
2. Do the same with high fives. What do you learn about your classmates through these simple forms of touch?
3. Experiment with a different style of handshake or high five.
4. How does this affect the way others perceive you?

Language of Touch

Practice 3: Physical Boundaries

Stand facing a partner. Experiment with your position relative to your partner.

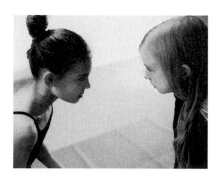

1. If you stand very close, how does it make you feel? Your partner?
2. If you stand far away, is it a different experience? In what way?

Discuss the ideal position in relationship to your partner that feels neither invasive nor standoffish.

Boundaries

3. How is that different for different groups within your class?
4. Is it different for members of the opposite sex?
5. Do boundaries change with acquaintances versus close friends?

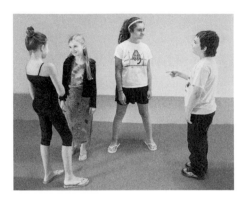

Comfortable Distance

In Touch Lessons

1. Huh Breath three times
2. Pursed lips: Sitting relaxed, purse your lips with an open space between the teeth.
   • Pursed lips inhale: Cooling
   a. Inhale through pursed lips; breath feels cool.
   b. Exhale through the nostrils.
   c. Repeat three times.
   • Pursed lips exhale: Lengthening.
   d. Inhale through the nose.
   e. Exhale through pursed lips; exhalation is long and slow.
   f. Repeat three times.

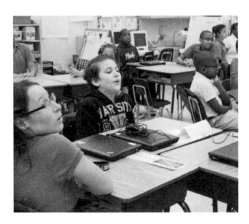

Pursed Lips

3. Rumbling Throat Breath
   a. Inhale through the relaxed open mouth.
   b. With your palm close to your mouth, exhale through the relaxed open mouth in a slow, soft, effortless stream; feel the warm breath on your palm.
   c. Repeat three times.
   d. Now close your mouth and remove your hand, but continue to breathe in the same way. Imagine that you are breathing in and out through your throat. Do you hear the soft rumbling sound deep in your throat?

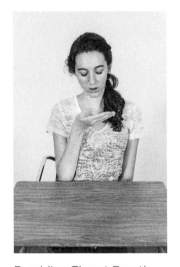

Rumbling Throat Breath

e. Repeat three times.

4. Folded Leaf variations

a. Chair Folded Leaf, strength variation: Sitting up tall, stretch your arms overhead. Inhale in the pose. With an exhalation, hinge forward, keeping your back long and straight. Inhale back upright and repeat.

b. Chair Folded Leaf, relaxed variation (see photo p. 242): Inhale and reach your arms up. Exhaling, slide your hands down your thighs as you lower your chest. Support your head with your hands or dangle your arms toward the ground.

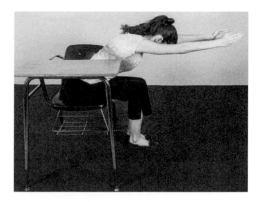

Folded Leaf Strength

c. In what ways do these variations of this posture feel different?

5. Partner poses back to back: How close is too close or just right when working with others?

a. Back-to-back Tree Pose: Stand back to back with your partner. Determine which leg you will stand on first, and keep the heel of your standing foot comfortably close to your partner's. Elevate the other foot, placing it above or below the knee. Bring your hands overhead and reach for your partner's hands. Clasp your palms together if you can, fingers touching your partner's.

b. Back-to-back Side Angle pose: Stand back to back with your partner, lightly touching. Together step one foot forward, bending your forward knee. When you are both ready, lift your arms out to the sides. Hold hands. With an exhalation, lower the hand of the forward knee down and the other up. Inhale and exhale. When you are both ready, straighten the bent knee and lift out of the posture. Repeat to the other side.

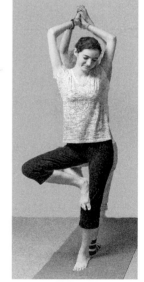

Back to Back Tree

Partner Side Angle Pose

6. Partner poses standing face to face: How do you touch others? Strong enough for support yet softly enough to do no harm?

a. Standing Twist: Facing your partner, each of you brings your right arm behind your back. With your left hand, reach across toward your partner's right hand and take hold. Ever so gently, twist your upper body away from your left hand. Can you feel how hard to pull? How much to let go?

b. Partner Down Dog: Stand facing your partner, holding hands. Slowly begin to back away from each other until your arms are stretched. Stabilize your feet under your hips as you stretch your back away from your partner. Communicate to be certain each partner is comfortable.

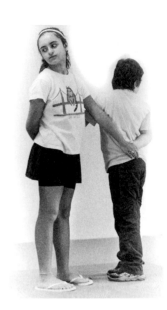
Standing Twist

c. Partner Up Dog: Face your partner, holding hands. Stand apart so that your arms are straight. Lean back, using your feet and back muscles, and look up with an inhalation. Signal your partner when you are ready to come out of the posture so you will both be ready. Walk toward each other and release hands.

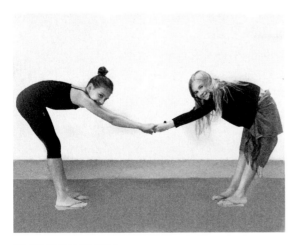
Partner Down Dog

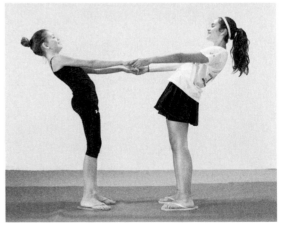
Partner Up Dog

7. Using touch: Neck release
   a. Neck rotations: Rotate your head to the right; notice how far you see to the right. Rotate your head to the left; notice how far you can see to the left.
   b. Scruff of the neck: Hold the scruff of your neck (where a cat holds her kittens) and gently nod "yes"; gently shake "no" (Bertherat & Bernstein, 1977). Release.
   c. Neck rotations: repeat the rotations, noticing if you can see farther in either direction.

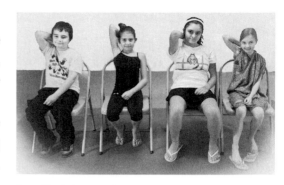

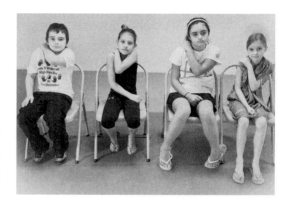

Scruff of the Neck

8. Using touch: Shoulder release
   a. Trapezius squeeze: Elevate the right shoulder. Grasp the right trapezius muscle with the left hand and let the shoulder gently drop. Slowly circle the shoulder in one direction; reverse. Release. Repeat on the opposite side.
   b. Shoulder circles: Relax the arms and circle the shoulders in one direction. Reverse.

Trapezius Squeeze

9. Using touch: Headache and sinus relief
   a. Sinus points: Smooth out the forehead with the fingertips. Apply gentle pressure with the flats of the fingers along the eyebrows.
   b. Temple press: Gently press the temple bones, in front of your ears. Hold or make small circles in each direction with your fingers.

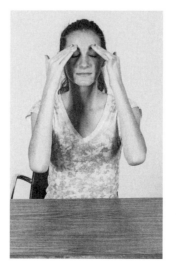

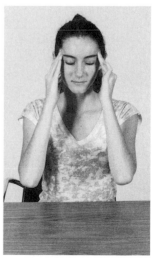

Sinus Points   Temple Press

c. Ear pull: Grasp the outer ear with your thumb and first finger. Very gently, pull the ears to release the facial muscles. Imagine the tension coming out the top of your head like steam.

d. Chin press: Rest your chin on your hands. Gently open your mouth without moving your hands; close. Repeat.

e. Yawn: Now yawn, drop your hands, and stretch your face and jaw.

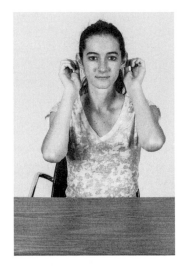

Ear Pull

10. Flower meditation: community connection. Each student is given a flower with many petals, such as a rose or daisy. Gaze at your flower, noticing its colors, its aroma, how delicate it feels against your skin. Now, begin to remove the petals gently, one at a time. Hold a petal and imagine that it is a very special gift.

a. Give the first petal to yourself.

b. Second, select a petal as a gift for the members of your family.

c. Next, a petal for your closest friends.

d. Then for your school community.

e. Next for your neighborhood community.

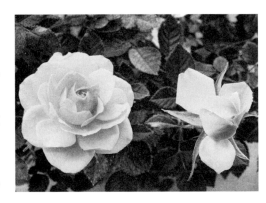

Flower Meditation

f. Now for your city, state, nation, earth, sun, stars, galaxy. . . .

g. Until you have given away all of the petals except one—save the last petal for yourself.

11. Huh Breath three times

Teacher Self-Care: Brief Routines for Classroom or Home

IF YOU HAVE a moment during your lunch break or prep time, you can release tension from your body without leaving your classroom.

Seated Self-Care

1. Huh Breath three times
2. Face points: Release sinus points by pressing gently around the orbit of the eyes with the pads of the fingers. Start with the eyebrows, then move out toward the temples, and back around the top of the cheekbones. Hold each point for a moment. Never

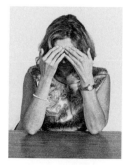 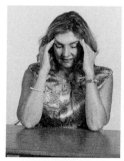 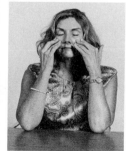

Eyebrow Press   Temple Press   Cheekbone Press

press into a soft area of the eye—only on bone; regulate pressure to your comfort.

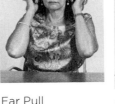

Ear Pull

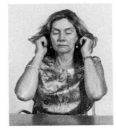

Trapezius Squeeze

3. Ear pull: Let your jaw go slack. Hold the cartilage of the widest portion of your ear between your forefinger (in front) and your thumb (in back). Ever so gently, pull the ear away from your face to relax the jaw.

4. Trapezius squeeze: Slide your right hand across your body and grasp your left trapezius muscle on top of your shoulder. With an inhalation, elevate your left shoulder; exhaling, lower your shoulder without releasing your grip. Slowly circle the shoulder in each direction (Bertherat & Bernstein, 1977). Release and repeat on the other side.

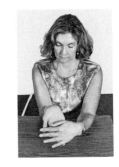

Wrist and Finger Extension

5. Wrist and finger extension: Use the right hand to gently stretch the palm and fingers of the left hand. Avoid with wrist or hand injury or if it causes discomfort.

6. Foot massage: Removing your shoe, use a tennis ball to massage the ball of your foot. Press lightly into the tennis ball—as long as it feels comfortable. Be sure to get the bottom of the toes, the full sole of the foot, and the heel. Repeat on the other side.

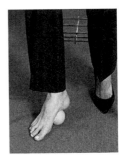

Foot Massage

7. Huh Breath three times

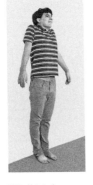

Wall Huh

Standing Self-Care: Wall Series

Kick off your shoes when you are alone in your classroom, and stretch out some tension. Or try these postures at home. Barefoot is recommended, but flat shoes are fine. Do not wear heels.

1. Wall Huh Breath three times: Standing with your back against the wall, slide your shoulders up the wall with an inhalation; exhaling with a "huh" sound, slide your shoulders back down.

2. Wall Chair: Stand with your back against the wall. Walk your feet about thigh length away from the wall as you bend your knees. Make certain that you are using your legs and the wall to support you. Do not go below thigh level. Be certain that your knees are comfortable and you've created no less than a 90-degree angle at your knees.

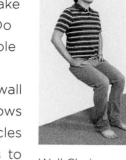

Wall Chair

a. Wall Cobra: Stand facing the wall with your palms on the wall, elbows bent. Begin to activate the muscles between your shoulder blades to bring them closer together and open your chest as you push slightly away from the wall. Bring the hands to chest level. Stay in position or walk your feet slightly farther from the wall to deepen the extension of the spine.

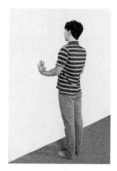

Wall Cobra

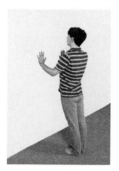

Wall Cobra Deeper

3. Wall Warrior 1: Stand facing the wall with your toes almost touching the wall and your hands in position for Wall Cobra. Step away from the wall with your right foot. Pressing away from the wall with your hands, bend your left knee gently toward the wall. Straighten your arms partially and keep your back comfortably upright. Engage your abdominal muscles to protect your lower back. Breathe. Step forward and change sides.

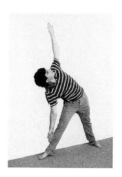

Wall Warrior 1

4. Wall Triangle: Stand with your back against the wall, feet wide apart, left foot straight, toes of the right foot pointing to the right. Elevate your arms to shoulder level, palms down. Turn to look over your right fingertips. Stay in this position or slide your right arm down the wall, the left arm up. Look straight ahead or past your left fingertips. Keep your head, back, shoulders, and the back of your hands on the wall for support. Slide up and repeat on the other side, going only so far as you are comfortable.

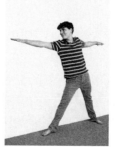

Wall Triangle 1

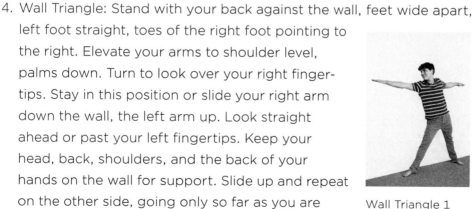

Wall Triangle

5. Wall Tree: Stand with your back against the wall and breathe. Shift your weight to your right foot and slide the sole of your left foot onto your inner shin. Bring your hands to your sternum; press the palms together to open your chest area. Release and repeat on the other side.

6. Wall Up Dog: Stand facing the wall and step one foot length back with both feet. Slide your arms up the wall to stretch the front of your body. Breathe deeply.

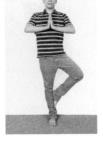   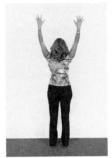

Wall Tree   Wall Up Dog

7. Wall Rag Doll: Standing with your back against the wall, bend your knees to relax your legs and back. Rest your hands on your thighs. Stay here or slide your arms slowly down your thighs and shins, lowering your upper body comfortably toward your shins. Do not hang down if you have high blood pressure, heart disease, seizure disorder, or it just doesn't feel right. Avoid immediately after eating.

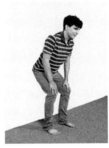   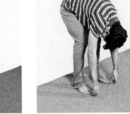

Wall Rag Doll 1   Wall Rag Doll

8. Wall Huh Breath three times

Home Care for Teachers

Here's a short routine for practice at home. It helps combat hours of sitting at a desk or computer. Wear loose, comfortable clothing and wait one hour after eating. As with any exercise regimen, it's always best to consult a physician and yoga educator before beginning, especially for those with conditions that require specific accommodations.

1. Half Airplane back strengthener: Lie on your belly face down with the arms straight and close to your sides, palms down. Press the tops of the feet, the front

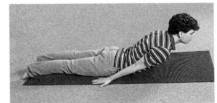

Airplane Back Strengthener

of the pelvis, and the hands firmly down. Inhale and lift the upper body only. Exhale and lower. Repeat.

2. Baby (Child's Pose): From hands and knees, gently sit back onto your feet, toes pointing backward. Lower your chest toward your thighs, your head on the ground, and your arms overhead or to your sides. If this is uncomfortable, support your chest and head with pillows or curl into a fetal position and rest on your side.

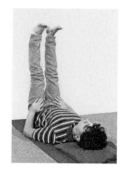

Baby (Child Pose)

3. Legs up the wall: Sit sideways close to the wall. Rolling onto your back, elevate your legs onto the wall, keeping your back fully on the ground. Be sure that your legs are completely supported by the wall. If it's too much of a stretch, place a rolled towel behind your knees, back away slightly from the wall, or come down and put your legs up over a chair instead. You may want a pillow under your head. Avoid if you have high blood pressure, heart disease, seizure disorder, after eating, or if just doesn't feel right.

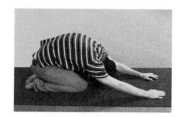

Legs Up the Wall

4. Knee hugs: On your back, hug your knees and rock from side to side. Hold the shin or backs of the thighs.

5. Open-armed supine twist: Lying on your back, lower your knees to the right and your head to the left. Open your arms out to the sides, below shoulder level. Breathe and relax. Reverse your knees and head. Avoid with spinal disc injuries.

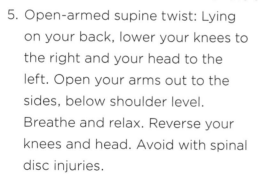

Knee Hugs

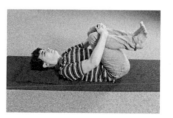

Open Armed Supine Twist

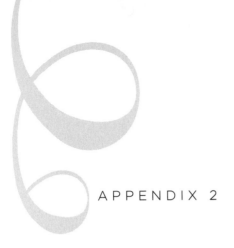

Home Practices for Students

T HE FOLLOWING IS a yoga routine that is safe for most students to practice independently. Wear loose, comfortable clothing and wait one hour after eating. As with any exercise regimen, it's always best to consult a physician and yoga educator before beginning, especially for those with conditions that require specific accommodations.

Seated

1. Three Huh Breaths: Sit cross-legged or in any position that's comfortable for you. Inhale, elevate the shoulders; exhale with a "huh" and let your shoulders drop.
2. Seated circles: With your hands on your knees, slowly circle the upper body without dropping your head. Reverse direction.

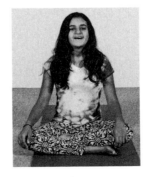
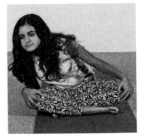

Huh Breath   Seated Circles

3. Butterfly knees: Bringing the soles of the feet together, gently open and close the knees. This can be done slowly, coordinating with the breathing—inhale knees up, exhale knees down. You may also move the knees more quickly as a warm-up.

4. Rock the Baby: Hold one foot in both hands or wrap your arms around your shin. Gently rock the hip as if you were lulling a baby to sleep. Switch legs.

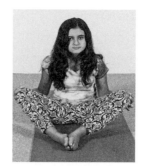
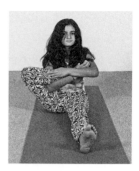

Butterfly Knees   Rock the Baby

5. Folded Leaf: Sit with your legs straight out in front of you. If you are uncomfortable, place rolled towels under your hips and beneath your knees. Reach your arms up high with an inhalation; exhaling, hinge forward from the hips without rounding your upper back. Lower your arms toward your legs. See if you can keep your back long without dropping your head. You may continue to move up and down, or rest and breathe in the lower position.

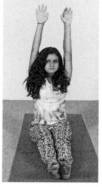
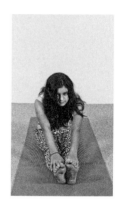

Folded Leaf Prep   Folded Leaf

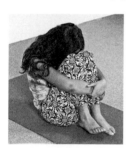

Seated Egg

6. Seated Egg (focusing inward): Sit with your arms around your knees, head tucked in, and feet relaxed on or off the floor. Notice your breathing in this quiet posture.

Hands and Knees

1. Happy Cat: From hands and knees, inhale and look up. Open your chest, and smile like a happy cat.

2. Angry Cat: Exhale and round your back toward the sky, like an angry cat. Repeat as many times as you like.

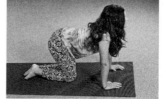
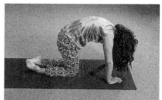

Happy Cat   Angry Cat

3. Balance Beam toe down: From hands and knees, straighten your left leg with the toe touching the ground behind you. Raise your right arm in front, looking past your fingertips. Release and switch sides.

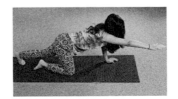

Balance Beam Toe Down

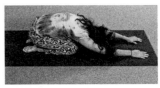

Baby

4. Baby: Push back and rest in baby posture (Child's Pose), with your arms overhead or palms up alongside your feet, whichever feels better. Let your head rest on the ground or use a cushion for support.

Belly

1. Belly rest: Rest on your belly and notice your breathing. Feel your body elevate away from the ground as you take in a breath; feel it sink back down as you exhale.

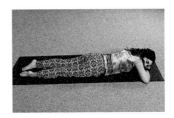

Belly Rest

2. Airplane: Stretch the arms out below shoulder level and turn your forehead to the ground. With an inhalation, elevate the arms, chest, and head (Half Airplane). Exhale down. If that was comfortable, repeat. If there is no back pain, inhale and raise the arms, head, and legs off the ground for Full Airplane. Exhale down. If comfortable, continue lifting up and down with the breath.

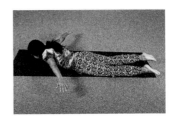

Airplane

3. Half Superman: Stretch both arms overhead, shoulder distance apart on the ground. Raise one arm and your head off the floor. Lower and repeat with the other arm. Now raise one leg only; lower and change legs. If all of these were comfortable, next time raise your right arm, head, and left leg off the floor. Lower. Now raise the left arm, head, and right leg. Lower. Repeat.

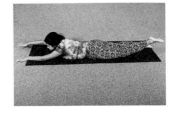

Half Superman

4. Baby: Push back and rest in baby or child's pose, with your arms overhead or by your feet, whichever feels better.

Back

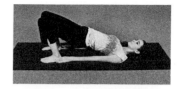

Bridge

1. Bridge: Come onto your back with your knees bent, feet hip distance apart, arms by your sides, palms down. Press the center of the back of your head, your hands, and feet into the ground. Elevate the hips with an inhalation; lower with an exhalation. Repeat.

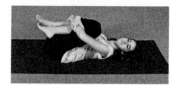

Knee Hugs

2. Knee hugs: Now hug your knees by wrapping your arms around or beneath your knees and rock from side to side.

3. Supine Open-Armed Twist: Lower your knees to the right, and open your arms out to your sides, below shoulder level. Turn your head in the opposite direction of your knees, toward your open left hand. Breathe. Switch head and knees to the opposite sides.

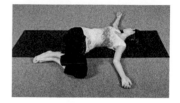

Supine Open Armed Twist

Standing

1. Fruit Picking: Standing up straight, imagine that you are picking your favorite fruit. Reach high for apples, low for strawberries, and to the sides for bananas.

2. Shake it out: Shake out your arms and legs. Have some fun!

3. Half Moon: Raise your arms up high and let them sway from side to side, forming a half moon on each side.

4. Willow Tree back bend: Like a willow tree whose branches blow in the breeze, let your arms sway all around you. A big wind blows your arms backward. Breathe and hold the posture.

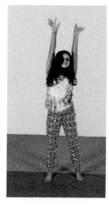 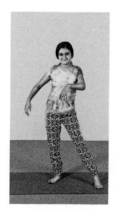 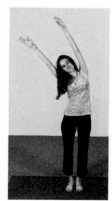 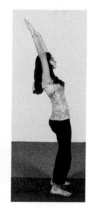

Fruit Picking   Shake It Out   Half Moon   Willow Tree Back Bend

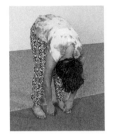

Rag Doll

5. Rag Doll: Gently fold forward at the hips, knees relaxed or bent, and hang your upper body like a rag doll. Breathe.

Supine Relaxation

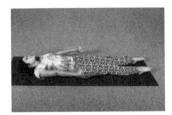

Tense and Relax

1. Tense and relax: Lying down on your back, tense your arms, legs, feet, hands and face. Now relax them all.

2. Float on a Cloud: Imagine that you are floating on a soft and fluffy cloud, made just for you. Allow your body to sink into this perfect cloud, knowing that you are safe and supported. This is how it feels to relax. Breathe in and out. Relax . . . relax . . . relax. Stay as long as you like.

3. Huh Breaths: Come up to a seated position and take three Huh Breaths to conclude your yoga session.

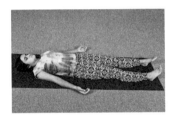

Float on a Cloud

Home Meditation: Bubbles

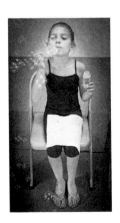

Bubbles

While blowing bubbles, let each bubble represent a thought or feeling that you would like to release. As you blow the bubbles, let go these thoughts and feelings.

Then find a comfortable seated position. Gaze at your open palms or close your eyes; observe your breathing, soft and steady. Each time a thought comes up, put it inside an imaginary bubble, and watch it float away. Let it go. Return your focus to your breathing or your open palms.

Start with 5 minutes of sitting. If you like, you may increase the time to 20 minutes by adding a minute each time you practice.

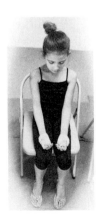

Home Meditation

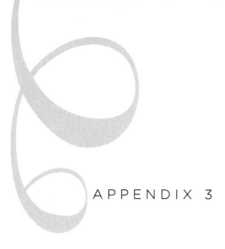

Personal Yoga Breaks: M.Y. Time (My Yoga Time)

Adapted with permission from *Yoga Therapy for Children with Autism and Special Needs* (Goldberg, 2013).

My Feelings, My Poses

Directions: Circle words that apply. Blanks may be filled in by student or with assistance.

Sometimes I feel tense

In my legs   My back

My shoulders   My face

My stomach   My mind

Other: _____

When _____ happens, I feel tense.

When I am tense, I feel _____ .

Sometimes I feel relaxed

    In my legs   My back

    My shoulders   My face

    My stomach   My mind

    Other: _____

    When _____ happens, I feel relaxed.

    When I am relaxed, I feel _____ .

Choose one pose that helps you feel relaxed:

    Bellows Breath

    Rag Doll

    Folded Leaf

    Breathing Tree

    Huh Breath

    Tense and Relax

    Other: _____

My favorite posture for having fun is:

    Shake It Out

    Fruit Picker

    Lion Breath

    Butterfly Hands

    Volcano

    Twister

    Other: _____

My favorite posture for feeling quiet is:

Floating on a Cloud

Counting Breath

Folded Leaf

Bellows Breath 2: Chin Tuck

Other: _____

My favorite postures for _____ are:

1. _____

2. _____

When things are just not going right, there is one pose that I can count on to make me feel better. This is My Yoga Time: MY TIME.

MY TIME pose is _____.

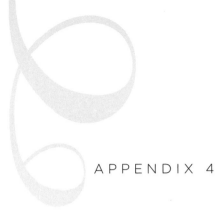

Warm-Ups and Cool-Down Routines for Physical Education

5-Minute Warm-Ups

1. Mountain pose: Stand straight and strong like a mountain, with the feet slightly apart and arms straight down by your sides.

2. Warrior 1 Heart Lift: Step the right foot forward, knee bent, into Warrior 1. Elevate the arms and sweep them overhead with a deep breath in. Exhale, release, and repeat on the other side.

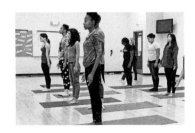

Mountain

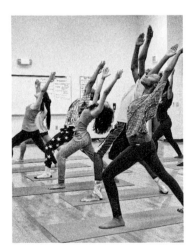

Warrior 1 Heart Lift

3. Down Dog: Come into table pose, on hands and knees. Walk or hop the feet back into down dog. Inhale and come up on the toes; exhale and lower the heels. Repeat twice more.

4. Up Dog: Glide the upper body forward on strong legs into Upward-Facing Dog. Breathe in position.

5. Dog Flow: Flow from Down Dog with an exhalation to Up Dog with an inhalation. Repeat as many times as is comfortable, to give the whole body a good stretch. Conclude in Down Dog.

6. Lunge Balance: From Down Dog, step the right foot forward and bring the back knee down into a lunge. Use the hands on the floor if needed. When it's comfortable, bring the palms together to open the chest and center you in this balance pose.

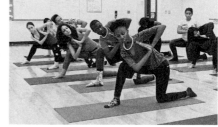

Down Dog

Up Dog

7. Side Angle Twist: From Lunge Balance with the palms together, rotate the upper body toward the bent knee. Deepen the twist by bringing the right arm in front of

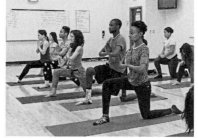

Lunge Balance

Side Angle Twist

the bent knee, palms pressed together. Return to center and step back into Warrior 1 and Down Dog. Repeat Lunge Balance and Side Angle Twist on the other side.

8. Mountain Pose

Now you are ready to continue with class.

5-Minute Cool-Down

1. Mountain Pose: Stand straight and strong like a mountain, with the feet slightly apart and arms straight down by your sides.

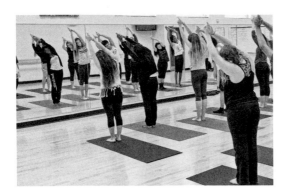

Lateral Flexion

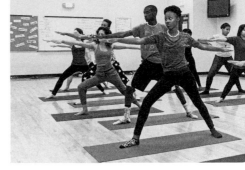

Warrior 2

2. Lateral Flexion: Interlace the fingers and straighten the forefingers, finger pads touching. Elevate both arms and lean to the right. Breathe and hold. Repeat to the left.

3. Warrior 2: Step the feet apart and turn the toes of both feet toward the right, keeping the body parallel to the yoga mat. Open the arms out to the sides and bend your right knee without shifting the weight to the right foot. Gaze past the right fingertips. Breathe. Reverse.

4. Triangle pose: With the feet spread wide, open the arms out to the side. Turn the toes of both feet to the left. Raise the right arm overhead as you lower the left arm toward your left shin. Try to keep your left arm and head in line with your upper arm. Come up and repeat to the right.

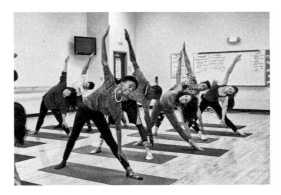

Triangle Pose

5. Upward Tree: Standing with the feet hip distance apart, shift the weight to the right foot. Keep your eyes focused on a point on the ground about 5 feet away, approximately your height. Slowly raise the left foot and place the sole of the foot inside your right

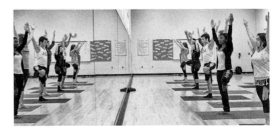

Upward Tree

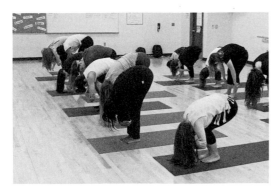

Bent Knee Rag Doll

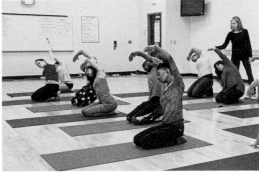

Hero Side Stretch

leg, below or above the knee. Slowly raise the open arms up overhead. Breathe. Release and repeat on the other side.

6. Bent-Knee Rag Doll: Bend your knees and allow your body to hang slowly down, arms dangling or holding the opposite elbow. Breathe.

7. Hero Side Stretch: Sit down on your heels. Elevate your left arm and lean to the right; breathe. Come back to center. Lift your right arm and lean to the left; breathe. Return to center.

8. Supine Twist: Lying on your back, bring your knees into your chest. Slowly lower the knees to one side. Open the arms to rest on the ground. Breathe in position. Lower the knees to the other side.

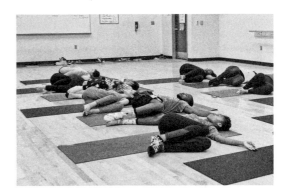

Supine Twist

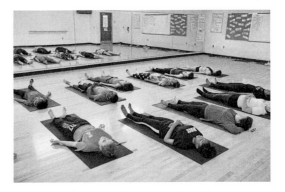

Deep Relaxation (Float on a Cloud)

9. Deep Relaxation (Float on a Cloud): Lie on your back with your arms and legs completely stretched out, surrendered into the ground. Scan your body and release any tension that you encounter. Follow the slow, steady

rhythm of your own breathing. Relax. (You may talk students through progressively tensing and relaxing their muscles, describe a calming scene, or just let them rest in this quiet place for a moment at the end of class.)

1-Minute Cool-Down Pose: Baby

If you have only a minute to relax, you can count on Baby to relax your body and mind.

Come onto your hands and knees. Sit back on the heels, allowing the toes to point back so you can rest your weight comfortably on the soles of the feet. Rest your head on the ground and your arms by your sides, palms up close to your feet. If this position is not comfortable, use a pillow beneath your head, or rest on your side curled into a ball.

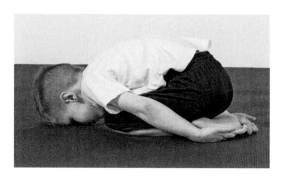

Baby

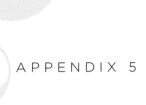

Core Strength Routine from NFL Player Jeremy Cain

I ASKED LONG SNAPPER Jeremy Cain of the National Football League to choose three postures that he has found especially helpful to increase core strength, balance, and focus. He selected the following postures:

Downward-Facing Dog: You can see the length through the whole back of his body in this pose, from his heels through his shoulders and arms. He is focused on his breathing in this posture. The combination of strength and flexibility is why Jeremy finds yoga so helpful to his game. When you practice this pose, keep a soft bend in your knees until you can keep the heels on the ground.

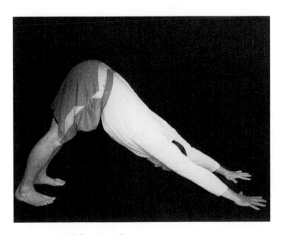

Downward Facing Dog

Upward-Facing Boat: This balance pose requires focus and core strength.

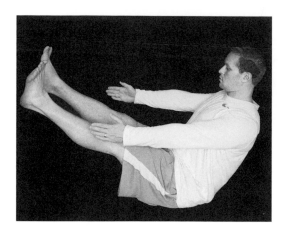

Upward Facing Boat

When attempting this pose, work first with bent knees. Straightening the legs requires strong abdominal and thigh muscles and exceptional balance.

Start with both feet on the floor, knees bent and close to the body. The first challenge is to sit upright on the sit bones without rolling back onto the tail bone. Raise the feet slightly off the ground, keeping all the muscles in the front of the body engaged, as well as those in the middle back. Slowly, straighten one knee, elevating the leg. Lower and switch legs. If this is comfortable, straighten both legs. Avoid this posture if there is lower back pain.

Crow: This is not a posture for beginners or those with wrist or shoulder injuries. Starting with a squat, the weight is shifted to the hands and arms. Each knee is tucked above the elbows, which are kept bent. Keeping a focal point for the eyes and mind is essential. Crow requires strength, flexibility, and balance—combining all the benefits of yoga.

Follow this routine with either Baby pose or the cool-down routine from Appendix 4.

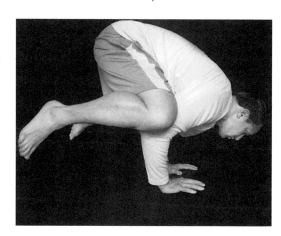

Crow

References

Abcarian, R. (2013). Yoga in public schools is exercise, not religion. *Los Angeles Times*. Retrieved from http://articles.latimes.com/2013/jul/01/local/la-me -ln-religious-objections-yoga-public-schools-20130701

Abdou, A. M., Higashiguchi, S., Horie, K., Kim, M., Hatta, H., & Yokogoshi, H. (2006). Relaxation and immunity enhancement effects of gamma-aminobutyric acid (GABA) administration in humans. *Biofactors, 26*(3), 201–208.

Administration for Children and Families. (2013). Child maltreatment 2013. Retrieved from https://www.acf.hhs.gov/sites/default/files/cb/cm2013.pdf

Alter, C. (2014, January 15). White House: Michelle Obama is picking up yoga. *Time.* Retrieved from http://swampland.time.com/2014/01/15/michelle -obama-is-picking-up-yoga/

American Psychological Association. (2014, February 11). American Psychological Association survey shows teen stress rivals that of adults. Retrieved from http://www.apa.org/news/press/releases/2014/02/teen-stress.aspx

Anxiety and Depression Association of America. (2016). Test Anxiety. Retrieved from http://www.adaa.org/living-with-anxiety/children/test-anxiety

Ayres, A. J. (1995.) *Sensory integration and the child*. Los Angeles, CA: Western Psychological Services.

Baird, T. (2014). Kripalu yoga in schools symposium 2014. Kripalu Center for Yoga and Health. Lenox, MA.

Beauchemin, J., Hutchins, T. L., & Patterson, F. (2008). Mindfulness meditation may lessen anxiety, promote social skills and improve academic performance among adolescents with learning disabilities. *Complementary Health Practice Review, 13*, 34–45.

Bertherat, T., & Bernstein, C. (1977). *The body has its reasons*. New York: Avon.

Biegel, G. M., Brown, K. W., Shapiro, S. L., & Schubert, C. M. (2009). Mindfulness-based stress reduction for the treatment of adolescent psychiatric outpatients: A randomized clinical trial. *Journal of Consulting and Clinical Psychology, 77*, 855–866.

Birdee, G. S., Yeh, G. Y., Wayne, P. M., Phillips, R. S., Davis, R. B., & Gardiner, P. (2009). Clinical applications of yoga for the pediatric population: A systematic review. *Academic Pediatrics, 9*(4), 212–220.

Black, L. I., Clarke, T. C., Barnes, P. M., Stussman, B. J., & Nahin, R. L. (2015). Use of complementary health approaches among children aged 4–17 years in the United States: National Health Interview Survey, 2007–2012. *National Health Statistics Reports*, no. 78, 1–19.

Blanchard, K., Lacinak, T., Thompkins, C., & Ballard, J. (2002). *Whale done! The power of positive relationships*. New York: Free Press.

Book, A., Costello, K., & Camilleri, J. A. (2013). Psychopathy and victim selection: The use of gait as a cue to vulnerability. *Journal of Interpersonal Violence, 28*, 2368–2383. doi:10.1177/0886260512475315

Branchi, I., D'Andrea, I., Fiore, M., Di Fausto, V., Aloe, L., & Alleva, E. (2006). Early social enrichment shapes social behavior and nerve growth factor and brain-derived neurotrophic factor levels in the adult mouse brain. *Biological Psychiatry, 60*, 690–696. doi:10.1016/j.biopsych.2006.01.005

Bremner, J., Elzinga, B., Schmahl, C., & Vermetten, E. (2008). Structural and functional plasticity of the human brain in posttraumatic stress disorder. *Progressive Brain Research, 167*, 171–186.

Bremner, J. D., Narayan, M., Anderson, E. R., Staib, L. H., Miller, H. L., & Charney, D. S. (2000). Hippocampal volume reduction in major depression. *American Journal of Psychiatry, 157*, 115–117.

Broderick, P. C., & Frank, J. L. (2014). Learning to BREATHE: An intervention to foster mindfulness in adolescence. *New Directions in Youth Development, 142*, 31–44.

Broderick, P. C., & Metz, S. (2009). Learning to BREATHE: A pilot trial of a mindfulness curriculum for adolescents. *Advances in School Mental Health Promotion, 2*, 35–46.

Brown, R., & Gerbarg, P. (2012). *The healing power of the breath: Simple techniques to reduce stress and anxiety, enhance concentration, and balance your emotions.* Boston: Shambhala.

Brown, R., Gerbarg, P., & Muskin, P. (2009). *How to use herbs, nutrients, and yoga in mental health care.* New York: Norton.

Butzer, B., Day, D., Potts, A., Ryan, C., Coulombe, S., Davies, B., Weidknecht, K., Ebert, M., Flynn, L., & Khalsa, S. B. S. (2015). Effects of a classroom-based yoga intervention on cortisol and behavior in second- and third-grade students: A pilot study. *Journal of Evidence-Based Complementary and Alternative Medicine, 20*, 41–49.

Butzer, B., Ebert, M., Telles, S., & Khalsa, S. B. S. (2015). School-based yoga programs in the United States: A survey. *Advances in Mind-Body Medicine, 29,* 18–26.

Butzer, B., & Flynn, L. (2016, April). *Research Repository: Yoga, Meditation and Mindfulness for Children, Adolescents and in Schools.* Retrieved from http://www.yoga4classrooms.com/supporting-research.

Cabot, E. L., Andrews, F. F., Coe, F. E., & Hill, M. (1918). The three sieves. In *A course in citizenship and patriotism* (pp. 103–104). Cambridge, MA: Houghton Mifflin. Retrieved from https://archive.org/details/acourseincitize01hillgoog

Cabral, P., Meyer, H. B., & Ames, D. (2011). Effectiveness of yoga therapy as a complementary treatment for major psychiatric disorders: A meta-analysis. *Primary Care Companion to CNS Disorders*, *13*(4), PCC.10r01068. Retrieved from http://www.psychiatrist.com/pcc/article/Pages/2011/v13n04/10r01068.aspx

Cauraugh, J. H., & Summers, J. J. (2005). Neural plasticity and bilateral movements: A rehabilitation approach for chronic stroke. *Progress in Neurobiology, 75*, 309–320.

Celebrities who swear by yoga can teach us a thing or two about balance. (2014). HuffPost Celebrity. Retrieved from http://www.huffingtonpost.com/2014/02/22/celebrities-love-yoga_n_4818678.html

Centeio, E., Whalen, L., Kulik, N., Thomas, E., & McCaughtry, N. (2015). Understanding stress and aggression behaviors among urban youth. *Journal of Yoga and Physical Therapy, 5*, 187. doi:10.4172/2157-7595.1000187

Center on the Developing Child at Harvard University. (2011). *Building the brain's "air traffic control" system: How early experiences shape the development of executive function. Working Paper No. 11.* Retrieved from http:// developingchild.harvard.edu/resources/building-the-brains-air-traffic -control-system-how-early-experiences-shape-the-development-of-execu tive-function/

Center on the Developing Child at Harvard University. (2015a). Executive function and self-regulation. Retrieved from http://developingchild.harvard.edu /key_concepts/executive_function/

Center on the Developing Child at Harvard University. (2015b). Supportive relationships and active skill-building strengthen the foundations of resilience: Working paper 13. Retrieved from http://www.developingchild.harvard.edu /resources/supportive-relationships-and-active-skill-building-strengthen -the-foundations-of-resilience/

Centers for Disease Control and Prevention. (2015a). Child abuse prevention. Retrieved from http://www.cdc.gov/features/healthychildren/

Centers for Disease Control and Prevention. (2015b). Healthy schools: Physical activity facts. Retrieved from http://www.cdc.gov/healthyschools/physical activity/facts.htm

Centers for Disease Control and Prevention. (2016). Child maltreatment prevention. Retrieved from http://www.cdc.gov/violenceprevention/childmaltreat ment/index.html

Chang, L. (Ed.). (2006). *Wisdom for the soul: Five millennia of prescriptions for spiritual healing.* Washington, DC: Gnosophia.

Children and Adults With Attention Deficit/Hyperactivity Disorder. (2015). Retrieved from http://www.chadd.org/Understanding-ADHD/About-ADHD .aspx

Children's Defense Fund. (2010, March). Children's Defense Fund mental health fact sheet. Retrieved from http://www.childrensdefense.org/library/data /mental-health-factsheet.pdf

Childress, T., & Cohen Harper, J. C. (Eds.). (2015). *Best practices for yoga in schools: Yoga service best practices guide* (Vol. 1). Atlanta: YSC-Omega.

Chopra, D., Malhotra, S., & Doraiswamy, P. M. (2015, June 21). Yoga and the brain: A vision of possibilities. *HuffPost Healthy Living.* Retrieved from http://

www.huffingtonpost.com/deepak-chopra/yoga-and-the-brain-a-visi
_b_7605504.html

Clarke, T. C., Black, L. I., Stussman, B. J., Barnes, P. M., & Nahin. R. L. (2015) Trends in the use of complementary health approaches among adults: United States, 2002-2012. *National Health Statistics Reports*, no. 79, 1–16.

Cleveland Clinic Foundation. (2014). Diaphragmatic breathing. Retrieved from http://my.clevelandclinic.org/health/diseases_conditions/hic_Understand ing_COPD/hic_Pulmonary_Rehabilitation_Is_it_for_You/hic_Diaphrag matic_Breathing

Coan, J. A., Schaefer, H. S., & Davidson, R. J. (2006). Lending a hand: Social regulation of the neural response to threat. *Psychological Science, 17*(12), 1032–1039.

Cole, R. (2007, August 28). Plumb perfect. *Yoga Journal*. Retrieved from http://www.yogajournal.com/article/practice-section/plumb-perfect/

Cole, R. (2008, December). Conditions for calm. *Yoga Journal*, 87–90.

Collaborative for Academic, Social, and Emotional Learning (CASEL). (2015). What is social and emotional learning? Retrieved from http://www.casel.org/social-and-emotional-learning/

Collins, D., & Goldberg, L. (2012, Winter). Evidenced-based practices in teaching self-calming to special needs children. Paper presented at Learning and the Brain 31st Conference, San Francisco, CA.

Conboy, L. A., Noggle, J. J., Frey, J. L., Kudesia, R. S., & Khalsa, S. B. S. (2013). Qualitative evaluation of a high school yoga program: Feasibility and perceived benefits. *Explore: The Journal of Science and Healing, 9*, 171–180. doi:10.1016/j.explore.2013.02.001

Cook-Cottone, C. P. (2015). Incorporating positive body image into the treatment of eating disorders: A model for attunement and mindful self-care. *Body Image, 14*, 158–167.

Cook-Cottone, C. P. (2016). The last word: Embodied self-regulation and mindful self-care in the prevention of eating disorders. *Eating Disorders: The Journal of Treatment and Prevention, 24*(1), 98–105. doi:10.1080/10640266.2015.1118954

Coulter, D. (2001). *Anatomy of hatha yoga*. Honesdale, PA: Body and Breath.

Court of Appeal. (2015, April 3). *Sedlock et al. v. Baird et al.* Fourth Appellate

District, Division One, State of California. Super. Ct. No. 37-2013-00035910 -CU-MC-CTL. Retrieved from https://www.yogaalliance.org/Portals/0/Ap pellate%20Opinion_04.03.15.pdf

Cousins, N. (1979). *Anatomy of an illness: As perceived by the patient*. New York: Norton.

Cullis, L. (2015). Yoga at the White House Easter egg roll. Leah Cullis. Retrieved from http://leahcullis.com/yoga-at-the-white-house/

Dennison, P., & Dennison, G. (1986). *Brain gym*. Glendale, CA: Edu-Kinesthetics.

Desbordes, G., Negi, L. T., Pace, T. W. W., Wallace, B. A., Raison, C. L., & Schwartz, E. L. (2012). Effects of mindful-attention and compassion medita- tion training on amygdala response to emotional stimuli in an ordinary, non- meditative state. *Frontiers in Human Neuroscience, 6*, 292. http://dx.doi .org/10.3389/fnhum.2012.00292

Desikachar, T. K. V. (1995). *The heart of yoga*. Rochester, VT: Inner Traditions.

Devi, N. J. (2007). *The secret power of yoga*. New York: Three Rivers.

Diamond, A. (2012). Activities and programs that improve children's executive functions. *Current Directions in Psychological Science, 21*, 335–341.

Diamond, M. C., Krech, D., & Rosenzweig, M. R. (1964). The effects of an enriched environment on the histology of the rat cerebral cortex. *Journal of Compara- tive Neurology, 123*, 111–119. doi:10.1002/cne.901230110

Doidge, N. (2007). *The brain that changes itself*. London: Penguin.

Douglass, L. (2010). Yoga in the public schools: Diversity, democracy and the use of critical thinking in educational debates. *Religion and Education, 37*(2), 162–174.

Duckworth, A. L., & Seligman, M. E. P. (2005). Self-discipline outdoes IQ in pre- dicting academic performance of adolescents. *Psychological Science, 16*(12), 939–944. doi:10.1111/j.1467-9280.2005.01641.x

Durlak, J. A., Weissberg, R. P., Dymnicki, A. B., Taylor, R. D., & Schellinger, K. B. (2011). The impact of enhancing students' social and emotional learning: A meta-analysis of school-based universal interventions. *Child Development, 82*, 405–432. Retrieved from http://static1.squarespace.com/static/513f 79f9e4b05ce7b70e9673/t/52e9d8e6e4b001f5c1f6c27d/1391057126694 /meta-analysis-child-development.pdf

Easwaran, E. (Trans.). (2007). *The Bhagavad Gita*. Berkley, CA: Nilgiri.

Engh, F. (2002). *Why Johnny hates sports*. Garden City Park, NY: Square One.

Ennis, C. D. (1999). Creating a culturally relevant curriculum for disengaged girls. *Sport, Education, and Society, 4*, 31–49.

Evans, G., Bullinger, M., & Hygge, S. (1998). Chronic noise exposure and physiological response: A prospective study of children living under environmental stress. *Psychological Science, 9*, 75–77.

Faherty, C. (2000). *Asperger's: What does it mean to me?* Arlington, TX: Future Horizons.

Faridi, S. (2014, June 24). Happy teaching, happy learning: 13 secrets to Finland's success. *Education Week*. Retrieved from http://www.edweek.org/tm/articles/2014/06/24/ctq_faridi_finland.html

Fears, N. (2014, December 14). Meditation program in California schools reduces violence and improves performance. *Inquisitr*. Retrieved from http://www.inquisitr.com/1717291/meditation-program-in-california-schools-reduces-violence-and-improves-performance/

Feuerstein, G. (1997). *The Shambala encyclopedia of yoga.* Boston: Shambala.

Feuerstein, G. (1998). *Yoga tradition.* Prescott, AZ: Hohm.

Field, T. (2011). Yoga clinical research review. *Complementary Therapies in Clinical Practice, 17*, 1–8.

Fishman, L., & Saltonstall, E. (2008). *Yoga for arthritis.* New York: Norton.

Flook, L., Smalley, S. L., Kitil, M. J., Dang, J., Cho, J., Kaiser-Greenland, S., Locke, J., & Kasari, C. (2010, April). A mindful awareness practice improves executive function in preschool children. *Journal of Applied School Psychology, 26*, 70–95. doi:10.1080/15377900903379125

Flynn, L. (2011). *Yoga 4 Classrooms activity card deck.* Dover, NH: Yoga 4 Classrooms.

Frank, J., Bose, B., & Schrobenhauser-Clonan, A. (2014). Effectiveness of a school-based yoga program on adolescent mental health, stress coping strategies, and attitudes toward violence: Findings from a high-risk sample. *Journal of Applied School Psychology, 30*(1), 29–49. Retrieved from http://www.tandfonline.com/loi/wapp20

Froeliger, B., Garland, E., & McClernon, F. J. (2012). Yoga meditation practitioners exhibit greater gray matter volume and fewer reported cognitive failures: Results of a preliminary voxel-based morphometric analysis. *Evidence-Based Complementary and Alternative Medicine*, 821307. doi:10.1155/2012/821307

Gage, F. (2003). Brain, repair yourself. *Scientific American, 289*(3), 46–53.

Galantino, M. L., Galbavy, R., & Quinn, L. (2008). Therapeutic effects of yoga for children: A systematic review of the literature. *Pediatric Physical Therapy, 20*(1), 66–80. doi:10.1097/PEP.0b013e31815f1208

Gandhi, M. K. (2000). *The Bhagavad Gita according to Gandhi.* Berkeley, CA: Berkeley Hills.

Gard, T., Noggle, J. J., Park, C. L., Vago, D. R., & Wilson, A. (2014). Potential self-regulatory mechanisms of yoga for psychological health. *Frontiers in Human Neuroscience, 8*, 770. http://doi.org/10.3389/fnhum.2014.00770

Gard, T., Taquet, M., Dixit, R., Hölzel, B. K., de Montjoye, Y.-A., Brach, N., . . . Lazar, S. W. (2014). Fluid intelligence and brain functional organization in aging yoga and meditation practitioners. *Frontiers in Aging Neuroscience, 6*, 76. http://doi.org/10.3389/fnagi.2014.00076

Gibran, K. (1998). *The prophet.* Oxford: One World.

Giedd, J. (2015). The amazing teen brain. *Scientific American, 312*(6), 32–37.

Gillen, L., & Gillen, J. (2008). *Yoga calm for children: Educating heart, mind, and body.* Portland, OR: Three Pebble.

Goldberg, L. (2004a). Creative relaxation: A yoga-based program for regular and exceptional student education. *International Journal of Yoga Therapy, 14*, 68–78.

Goldberg, L. (2004b). *Creative Relaxation: Yoga for children* [DVD]. Margate, FL: Relaxation Now.

Goldberg, L. (2011). *Creative Relaxation: Yoga therapy for children with autism and special needs manual* (rev. ed.). Margate, FL: Relaxation Now.

Goldberg, L. (2013). *Yoga therapy for children with autism and special needs.* New York: Norton.

Goldberg, L., Miller, S., Collins, D., & Morales, D. (2006). *S.T.O.P. and relax: Instructor's manual.* Margate, FL: STOP and Relax.

Goldin, P. R., & Gross, J. J. (2010). Effects of mindfulness-based stress reduction (MBSR) on emotion regulation in social anxiety disorder. *Emotion, 10*(1), 83–91.

Goleman, D. (2013). *Focus: The hidden driver of excellence.* New York: Harper-Collins.

Gothe, N. P., Kramer, A. F., & McAuley, E. (2014). The effects of an 8-week hatha yoga intervention on executive function in older adults. *Journals of Gerontol-*

ogy, Series A: Biological Sciences and Medical Sciences, 69(9), 1109–1116. doi:10.1093/gerona/glu095.

Gothe, N., Pontifex, M. B., Hillman, C. H., & McAuley, E. (2013). The acute effects of yoga on executive function. *Journal of Physical Activity and Health, 10*(4), 488–495.

Grandin, T. (2006). *Thinking in pictures.* New York: Vintage.

Greater Good Science Center. (2015). What is mindfulness? Retrieved from http://greatergood.berkeley.edu/topic/mindfulness/definition

Greenberg, M., & Harris, A. R. (2011). Nuturing mindfulness in children and youth: Current state of research. *Child Development Perspectives, 6,* 161–166. doi:10.1111/j.1750-8606.2011.00215.x

Greenberg, M. T., Weissberg, R. P., O'Brien, M. U., Zins, J. E., Fredericks, L., Resnik, H., & Elias, M. J. (2003). Enhancing school-based prevention and youth development through coordinated social, emotional, and academic learning. *American Psychologist, 58,* 466–474.

Hancock, L. (2011, September). Why are Finland's schools successful? *Smithsonian.* Retrieved from http://www.smithsonianmag.com/innovation/why-are -finlands-schools-successful-49859555/?no-ist

Hannaford, C. (2005). *Smart moves: Why learning is not all in your head* (rev. ed.). Salt Lake City, UT: Great River.

Hansen, D. M., Larson, R. W., & Dworkin, J. B. (2003). What adolescents learn in organized youth activities: A survey of self-reported developmental experiences. *Journal of Research on Adolescence, 13,* 25–55.

Hatfield, E., Cacioppo, J. L., & Rapson, R. L. (1993). Emotional contagion. *Current Directions in Psychological Sciences, 2,* 96–99.

Heart Math Institute. (2016). Heart brain communication. Retrieved from https:// www.heartmath.org/research/science-of-the-heart/heart-brain-commu nication/

Heid, M. (2014, November 19). You asked: Does laughing have real health benefits? *Time.* Retrieved from http://time.com/3592134/laughing-health-benefits/

Heil, E. (2014, June 4). Hillary Clinton dishes on Monica, 2016 and yoga in People mag. *Washington Post.* Retrieved from https://www.washingtonpost.com /news/reliable-source/wp/2014/06/04/hillary-clinton-dishes-on-monica -2016-and-yoga-in-people-mag/

Hillman, C., Buck, S., Themanson, J., Pontifex, M., & Castelli, D. (2009). Aerobic fitness and cognitive development: Event-related brain potential and task performance indices of executive control in preadolescent children. *Developmental Psychology, 45*, 114–129.

Hillman, C., Erickson, K., & Kramer, A. (2008). Be smart, exercise your heart: Exercise effects on brain and cognition. *Nature Reviews Neuroscience, 9*, 58–65.

Hillman, C., Motl, R., Pontifex, M., Posthuma, D., Stubbe, J., Boomsma, D., & de Geus, E. (2006). Exercise appears to improve brain function among younger people. *Health Psychology, 25*, 678–687.

Holloway, M. (2003). The mutable brain. *Scientific American, 289*(3), 78–85.

Hölzel, B. K., Carmody, J., Evans, K. C., Hoge, E. A., Dusek, J. A., Morgan, L., . . . Lazar, S. W. (2010). Stress reduction correlates with structural changes in the amygdala. *Social Cognitive and Affective Neuroscience, 5*(1), 11–17. http://doi.org/10.1093/scan/nsp034

Hölzel, B. K., Carmody, J., Vangel, M., Congleton, C., Yerramsetti, S. M., Gard, T., & Lazar, S. W. (2011). Mindfulness practice leads to increases in regional brain gray matter density. *Psychiatry Research, 191*(1), 36–43. http://doi.org/10.1016/j.pscychresns.2010.08.006

House, K. (2014, October 14). In "mindful studies" class, Wilson High School students learn to cope with teenage stress. *The Oregonian*. Retrieved from http://www.oregonlive.com/portland/index.ssf/2014/10/in_mindful_studies_class_wilso.html

Huang, Z. J., Kirkwood, A., Pizzorusso, T., Porciatti, V., Morales, B., Bear, M. F., Maffei, L., & Tonegawa, S. (1999). BDNF regulates the maturation of inhibition and the critical period of plasticity in mouse visual cortex. *Cell, 98*, 739–755.

Huppert, F. A., & Johnson, D. M. (2010). A controlled trial of mindfulness training in schools: The importance of practice for an impact on well-being. *Journal of Positive Psychology, 5*(4), 264–274.

Hyde, A. (2012). The yoga in schools movement: Using standards for educating the whole child and making space for teacher self-care. In J. A. Gorlewski, B. J. Porfilio, & D. A. Gorlewski (Eds.), *Using standards and high-stakes testing for students: Exploiting power with critical pedagogy*. New York: Peter Lang.

Iacoboni, M. (2008). *Mirroring people*. New York: Farrar, Straus and Giroux.

International Association of Yoga Therapists. (2012). Educational Standards for the Training of Yoga Therapists. Retrieved from http://www.iayt.org/development_Vx2/IAYT_Standards_7%201%2012%20.pdf

Iyengar, B. K. S. (1998). *Light on the yoga sutras of Patanjali*. San Francisco: Thorsons.

Iyengar, B. K. S. (2001). *Yoga: The path to holistic health*. London: Dorling Kindersley.

Jacobson, E. (1934). *You must relax*. New York: Whittlesey House.

Jaeggi, S. M., Buschkuehl, M., Jonides, J., & Perrig, W. J. (2008). Improving fluid intelligence with training on working memory. *Proceedings of the National Academy of Sciences of the United States of America, 105*(19), 6829–6833. http://doi.org/10.1073/pnas.0801268105

Janzen, J. (1996). *Understanding the nature of autism*. San Antonio, TX: Therapy Skill Builders.

Jennings, P. (2015). *Mindfulness for teachers*. New York: Norton.

Jennings, P. A., Snowberg, K. E., Coccia, M. A., & Greenberg, M. T. (2012). Refinement and evaluation of the CARE for Teachers program. In M. Greenberg (Chair), *Teachers' growth during targeted SEL professional development and SEL program implementation: An international perspective*. Symposium conducted at the annual meeting of the American Education Research Association, Vancouver, BC.

Jensen, E. (2008). *Brain-based learning: The new paradigm of teaching*. Thousand Oaks, CA: Corwin.

Jensen, F. (2015). *The teenage brain*. New York: Harper Collins.

Jerath, R., Crawford, M. W., Barnes, V. A., & Harden, K. (2015). Self-regulation of breathing as a primary treatment for anxiety. *Applied Psychophysiology and Biofeedback, 40*, 107–115. doi:10.1007/s10484-015-9279-8

Johnson, A. (2014). Kripalu yoga in schools symposium 2014. Kripalu Center for Yoga and Health. Lenox, MA

Jotika, U., & Dhamminda, U. (Trans.). (1986). *Maha Sattipatana sutta: The greater discourse on steadfast mindfulness of the Buddha*. Maymyo, Burma: Migadavun Monastery. Retrieved from http://www.buddhanet.net/pdf_file/mahasati.pdf

Kabat-Zinn, J. (1994). *Wherever you go, there you are: Mindfulness meditation in everyday life*. New York: Hyperion.

Kabat-Zinn, J. (1996). Mindfulness meditation: What it is, what it isn't, and its role in health care and medicine. In Y. Haruki, Y. Ishii, & M. Suzuki (Eds.), *Comparative and psychological study on meditation* (pp. 161–169). Netherlands: Eburon.

Keltner, D. (2009). *Born to be good.* New York: Norton.

Khalsa, S. B. (2004). Treatment of chronic insomnia with yoga: A preliminary study with sleep-wake diaries. *Applied Psychophysiology and Biofeedback, 29*(4), 269–278. Retrieved from http://www.ncbi.nlm.nih.gov/pubmed/1570 7256

Khalsa, S. B., Hickey-Schultz, L., Cohen, D., Steiner, N., & Cope, S. (2012). Evaluation of the mental health benefits of yoga in a secondary school: A preliminary randomized controlled trial. *Journal of Behavioral Health Services and Research, 39,* 80–90.

Khalsa, S. B., Shorter, S. M., Cope, S., Wyshak, G., & Sklar, E. (2009). Yoga ameliorates performance anxiety and mood disturbance in young professional musicians. *Applied Psychophysiology and Biofeedback, 34,* 279–289.

Khalsa, S. S., & Butzer, B. (2016). Yoga in school settings: a research review. *Annals of the New York Academy of Sciences.* doi: 10.1111/nyas.13025

Khalsa, S. P. K. (1996). *Kundalini yoga: The flow of eternal power.* New York: Penguin.

Kirkwood, G., Rampes, H., Tuffrey, V., Richardson, J., Pilkington, K., & Ramaratnam, S. (2005). Yoga for anxiety: A systematic review of the research. *British Journal of Sports Medicine, 39*(12), 884–891.

Kranowitz, C. S. (2005). *The out-of-sync child.* New York: Penguin.

Kripalu yoga in the schools curriculum. (2015). Kripalu Center for Yoga and Health. Stockbridge, MA.

Kumaran, D., (2008). Short-term memory and the human hippocampus. *Journal of Neuroscience, 28*(15), 3837–3838. Retrieved from http://www.jneurosci .org/content/28/15/3837.full.pdf+html

Lazar, S. W., Kerr, C. E., Wasserman, R. H., Gray, J. R., Greve, D. N., Treadway, M. T., . . . Fischl, B. (2005). Meditation experience is associated with increased cortical thickness. *NeuroReport, 16*(17), 1893–1897.

LeDoux, J. E. (1996). *The emotional brain.* New York: Simon and Schuster.

LeShan, L. (1974). *How to meditate.* Boston: Little, Brown.

Liehr, P., & Diaz, N. (2010). A pilot study examining the effects of mindfulness on depression and anxiety for minority children. *Archives of Psychiatric Nursing, 24*, 69–71.

Lupien, S. J., McEwen, B. S., Gunnar, M. R., & Heim, C. (2009). Effects of stress throughout the lifespan on the brain, behaviour and cognition. *Nature Reviews Neuroscience, 10*, 434–445.

Madigan, J. B. (2009). *Action based learning.* Murphy, TX: Building Better Brains Through Movement.

Maguire, E. A., Gadian, D. G., Johnsrude, I. S., Good, C. D., Ashburner, J., Frackowiak, R. S. J., & Frith, C. D. (2000). Navigation-related structural change in the hippocampi of taxi drivers. *Proceedings of the National Academy of Sciences of the United States of America, 97*(8), 4398–4403.

Marie, D., Wyshak, G., & Wyshak, G. H. (2008). Yoga prevents bullying in school. Calming Kids. Retrieved from http://www.calmingkidsyoga.org/Gifs/Yoga PreventsBullyingInSchool.pdf

Maslow, A. (1999). *Toward a psychology of being* (3rd ed.). New York: Wiley.

McCall, T. (2007). *Yoga as medicine.* New York, NY: Bantam-Dell.

McCorry, L. K. (2007). Physiology of the autonomic nervous system. *American Journal of Pharmaceutical Education, 71*(4), 78.

McEwen, B. (2002). *The end of stress as we know it.* New York: Dana.

Medina, J. (2008). *Brain rules: 12 principles for surviving and thriving at work, home, and school.* Seattle, WA: Pear Press.

Medina, J. (2012). *Brain rules: Exercise.* Seattle, WA: Pear Press. Retrieved from http://www.brainrules.net/exercise

Medina, J. (2014). *Brain rules (updated and expanded): 12 principles for surviving and thriving at work, home, and school* (2nd ed.). Seattle, WA: Pear Press.

Mendelson, T., Greenberg, M., Dariotis J., Gould, L., Rhoades, B., & Leaf, P. (2010). Feasibility and preliminary outcomes of a school-based mindfulness intervention for urban youth. *Journal of Abnormal Child Psychology, 38*, 985–994. doi:10.1007/s10802-010-9418-x

Mendelson, T., Dariotis, J., Gould, L., Smith, A. S. R., Atman, A., Smith, A. A., . . . Greenberg, M. (2013). Implementing mindfulness and yoga in urban schools: A community-academic partnership. *Journal of Children's Services, 8*(4), 276–291.

Merkel, D. L. (2013). Youth sport: Positive and negative impact on young athletes. *Open Access Journal of Sports Medicine, 4,* 151–160. http://doi.org /10.2147/OAJSM.S33556

Merritt, E. G., Wanless, S. B., Rimm-Kaufman, S. E., Cameron, C., & Peugh, J. L. (2012). The contributions of teachers' emotional support to children's social behaviors and self-regulatory skills in first grade. *School Psychologists Review, 41*(2), 141–159.

Mindful Practices. (2015). SEL research. Retrieved from http://www.mindful practicesyoga.com/about/research

Moffitt, T. E., Arseneault, L., Belsky, D., Dickson, N., Hancox, R. J., Harrington, H., . . . Caspi, A. (2011). A gradient of childhood self-control predicts health, wealth, and public safety. *Proceedings of the National Academy of Sciences of the United States of America, 108*(7), 2693–2698. doi:10.1073/pnas. 1010076108

Morin, A. (2014, November 23). 7 scientifically proven benefits of gratitude that will motivate you to give thanks year-round. *Forbes.* Retrieved from http:// www.forbes.com/sites/amymorin/2014/11/23/7-scientifically-proven -benefits-of-gratitude-that-will-motivate-you-to-give-thanks-year-round/

Muktibodhananda, S. (2001). *Hatha yoga pradipika.* Mungar, India: Yoga Publica- tions Trust.

Naropa University. (2015). About Naropa. Retrieved from http://www.naropa .edu/about-naropa/index.php

National Center for Complementary and Integrative Health. (2013, June). Yoga for health. Retrieved from https://nccih.nih.gov/health/yoga/introduction. htm

National Center for Complementary and Integrative Health. (2015, February 10). Nationwide survey reveals widespread use of mind and body practices. Retrieved from https://nccih.nih.gov/news/press/02102015mb

National Center for Health Statistics. (2012). *Health, United States, 2011: With special feature on socioeconomic status and health.* Hyattsville, MD: U.S. Department of Health and Human Services.

Norman, K. R. (1997). *A philological approach to buddhism: The Bukkyo Dendo Kyokai Lectures 1994.* London: School of Oriental and African Studies, Uni- versity of London.

Panksepp, J. (2007). Can play diminish ADHD and facilitate the construction of the social brain? *Journal of the Canadian Academy of Child and Adolescent Psychiatry, 16*(2), 57–66.

Panksepp, J. (2008). Play, ADHD and the construction of the social brain: Should the first class each day be recess? *American Journal of Play, 1*, 55–79.

Parker, A. E., Kupersmidt, J. B., Mathis, E. T., Scull, T. M., & Sims, C. (2014). The impact of mindfulness education on elementary school students: Evaluation of the Master Mind program. *Advances in School Mental Health Promotion, 7*(3), 184–204.

Pascual-Leone, A., Amedi, A., Fregni, F., & Merabet, L. B. (2005). The plastic human brain cortex. *Annual Review of Neuroscience, 28*, 377–401.

Paul, R. (2004). *The yoga of sound.* Novato, CA: New World Library.

Pearson, Ed. (2014). The learning curve 2014 Report Index. Retrieved from http://thelearningcurve.pearson.com/reports/the-learning-curve-report-2014

Peck, H. L., Kehle, T. J., Bray, M. A., & Theodore, L. A. (2005). Yoga as an intervention for children with attention problems. *School Psychology Review, 34*(3), 415–424.

Perry, B. (2015). Keep the cool in school: Self-regulation—the second core strength. Scholastic. Retrieved from http://www.scholastic.com/teachers/article/keep-cool-school-self-regulation-second-core-strength

Philippot, P., Chapelle, G., & Blairy, S. (2002). Respiratory feedback in the generation of emotion. *Cognition and Emotion, 16*, 605–627.

Piper, W. (1976). *The little engine that could.* New York: Platt and Munk.

Pittman, C., & Karle, E. (2015). *Rewire your anxious brain: How to use the neuroscience of fear to end anxiety, panic, and worry.* Oakland, CA: New Harbinger.

Pontifex, M. B., Hillman, C. H., Fernhall, B., Thompson, K. M., & Valentini, T. A. (2009). The effect of acute aerobic and resistance exercise on working memory. *Medicine and Science in Sports and Exercise, 41*(4), 927–934. doi:10.1249/MSS.0b013e3181907d69

Pontifex, M. B., Saliba, B. J., Raine, L. B., Picchietti, D. L., & Hillman, C. H. (2013). Exercise improves behavioral, neurocognitive, and scholastic performance in children with attention-deficit/hyperactivity disorder. *Journal of Pediatrics, 162*(3), 543–545.

Porges, S. (2005). The vagus: A mediator of behavioral and psychological features associated with autism. In M. Bauman & T. Kemper (Eds.), *The neurobiology of autism* (pp. 65–78). Baltimore, MD: Johns Hopkins University Press.

Porges, S. (2011). *The polyvagal theory: Neurophysiological foundations of emotions, attachment, communication, and self-regulation.* Norton Series on Interpersonal Neurobiology. New York: Norton.

Powell, L., Gilchrist, M., & Stapley, J. (2008). A journey of self-discovery: An intervention involving massage, yoga and relaxation for children with emotional and behavioural difficulties attending primary schools. *European Journal of Special Needs Education, 23*(4), 403–412.

Prabhavananda, S., & Isherwood, C. (1981). *How to know God: The yoga aphorisms of Patanjali.* Hollywood, CA: Vedanta.

Radhakrishna, S. (2010). Application of integrated yoga therapy to increase imitation skills in children with autism spectrum disorder. *International Journal of Yoga, 3*, 26–30.

Rama, S. (1982). *Enlightenment without God* (Mandukya Upanishad). Honesdale, PA: Himalayan Institute.

Ramon y Cajal, S. (1894). The Croonian lecture: La fine structure des centres nerveux. *Proceedings of the Royal Society of London, 55*, 444–468.

Ratey, J., with Hagerman, E. (2008). *Spark: The revolutionary new science of exercise and the brain.* Boston: Little, Brown.

Rennecke, A. (2015, August 17). Melrose football finding yoga classes helpful. *St. Cloud Times.* Retrieved from http://www.sctimes.com/story/sports/high-school/2015/08/17/rennecke-melrose-football-finding-yoga-classes-helpful/31845221/

Rideout, V. J., Foehr, U. G., & Roberts, D. F. (2010). Generation M2: Media in the lives of 8- to 18-year-olds. Menlo Park, California: Henry J. Kaiser Family Foundation. Retrieved from https://kaiserfamilyfoundation.files.wordpress.com/2013/01/8010.pdf

Robin, M. (2009). *A handbook for yogasana teachers.* Tucson, AZ: Wheatmark.

Rocha, K. K., Ribeiro, A. M., Rocha, K. C., Sousa, M. B., Albuquerque, F. S., Ribeiro, S., & Silva, R. H. (2012). Improvement in physiological and psychological parameters after 6 months of yoga practice. *Consciousness and Cognition, 21*(2), 843–850. doi:10.1016/j.concog.2012.01.014

Rosen, R. (2002, May–August). Q & A: Headstand and high blood pressure. *Yoga*

Studies. Retrieved from http://www.iayt.org/Publications_Vx2/news/news2 .aspx

Ross, A., & Thomas, S. (2010). The health benefits of yoga and exercise: A review of comparison studies. *Journal of Alternative and Complementary Medicine, 16*(1), 3–12. doi:10.1089/acm.2009.0044

Roth, L. (2014, October 13). Schools add yoga to help students unwind. *Orlando Sentinel.* Retrieved from http://www.orlandosentinel.com/features/educa tion/os-schools-yoga-pe-students-20141013-story.html

Ryan, T. (2012). *A mindful nation: How a simple practice can help us reduce stress, improve performance, and recapture the American spirit.* Carlsbad, CA: Hay House.

Saltzman, A. (2014). *A still quiet place.* Oakland, CA: Harbinger.

Sanford, M. (2006). *Waking.* Chicago, IL: Rodale.

Sanford, M. (2008). Matthew's vision. Retrieved from http://matthewsanford .com/content/matthews-vision

Sapolsky, R. (2003). Taming stress. *Scientific American, 289*(3), 86–95.

Schilling, E. A., Aseltine, R. H., Jr., & Gore, S. (2007). Adverse childhood experiences and mental health in young adults: A longitudinal survey. *BMC Public Health, 7,* 30. doi:10.1186/1471-2458-7-30

Schonert-Reichl, K. A., & Lawlor, M. S. (2010). The effects of a mindfulness-based education program on pre- and early adolescents' well-being and social and emotional competence. *Mindfulness, 1*(3), 137–151.

Scime, M., & Cook-Cottone, C. (2008). Primary prevention of eating disorders: A constructivist integration of mind and body strategies. *International Journal of Eating Disorders, 41*(2), 134–142.

Scime, M., Cook-Cottone, C., Kane, L., & Watson, T. (2006). Group prevention of eating disorders with fifth-grade females: Impact on body dissatisfaction, drive for thinness, and media influence on eating disorders. *Journal of Treatment and Prevention, 14*(2), 143–155. doi:10.1080/10640260500403881

Seidman, M. D., & Standring, R. T. (2010). Noise and quality of life. *International Journal of Environmental Research and Public Health*, *7*(10), 3730–3738. doi:10.3390/ijerph7103730

Selye, H. (1974). *Stress without distress.* New York: Signet.

Sequeira, S., & Ahmed, M. (2012). Meditation as a potential therapy for autism: A review. *Autism Research and Treatment, 2012.* doi:10.1155/2012/835847

Serwacki, M., & Cook-Cottone, C. (2012). Yoga in the schools: A systematic review of the literature. *International Journal of Yoga Therapy, 22*, 101–109.

Shannahoff-Khalsa, D. (2010). *Kundalini yoga meditation for complex psychiatric disorders: Techniques specific for treating the psychoses, personality, and pervasive developmental disorders.* New York: Norton.

Shelov, D. V., Suchday, S., & Friedberg, J. P. (2009). A pilot study measuring the impact of yoga on the trait of mindfulness. *Behavioural and Cognitive Psychotherapy, 37*(5), 595–598. doi:http://dx.doi.org/10.1017/S1352465809990361

Siegel, D. J. (2007). *The mindful brain: Reflection and attunement in the cultivation of well-being.* New York: Norton.

Siegel, D. J. (2011). *The whole-brain child: 12 revolutionary strategies to nurture your child's developing mind.* New York, NY: Delacorte Press.

Siegel, D. J. (2013). *Brainstorm: The power and purpose of the teenage brain.* New York: Penguin.

Silcox, K. (2014, October 14). Why do we set intentions in yoga? *Yoga Journal.* Retrieved from http://www.yogajournal.com/article/history-of-yoga/qa-set-intentions-yoga/

Simons, D. J., & Chabris, C. F. (1999). Gorillas in our midst: Sustained inattentional blindness for dynamic events. *Perception, 28*, 1059–1074.

Simons, D. J., & Chabris, C. F. (2010). *The invisible gorilla, and other ways our intuitions deceive us.* New York: Crown.

Singer, T., Critchley, H. D., & Preuschoff, K. (2009). A common role of insula in feelings, empathy and uncertainty. *Trends in Cognitive Sciences, 13*(8), 334–340. doi:10.1016/j.tics.2009.05.001

Slovacek, S. P., Tucker, S. A., & Pantoja, L. (2003). *Study of the Yoga Ed. program at the Accelerated School.* Los Angeles: Program Evaluation and Research Collaborative, Charter College of Education.

Sparrowe, L., & Walden, P. (2004). *Yoga for healthy bones: A woman's guide.* Boston: Shambala.

Spence, J. (2015). Kripalu yoga in schools symposium 2015. Kripalu Center for Yoga and Health. Lenox, MA

Sternberg, R. J. (2008). Increasing fluid intelligence is possible after all. *Proceedings of the National Academy of Sciences of the United States of America, 105*, 6791–6792. doi:10.1073/pnas.0803396105

Strauss, V. (2014, December 3). A therapist goes to middle school and tries to sit still and focus. *Washington Post.* Retrieved from http://www.washington post.com/blogs/answer-sheet/wp/2014/12/03/a-therapist-goes-to -middle-school-and-tries-to-sit-still-and-focus-she-cant-neither-can-the -kids/

Streeter, C., Gerbarg, P. L., Saper, R. B., Ciraulo, D. A., & Brown, R. P. (2012). Effects of yoga on the autonomic nervous system, gamma-aminobutyric-acid, and allostasis in epilepsy, depression, and post-traumatic stress disorder. *Medical Hypotheses, 78*, 571–579.

Streeter, C., Jensen, J., Perlmutter, R., Cabral, H., Tian, H., Terhune, D., . . . Renshaw, P. F. (2007). Yoga asana sessions increase brain GABA levels: A pilot study. *Journal of Alternative and Complementary Medicine, 13*, 419–426.

Streeter, C., Whitfield, T. H., Owen, L., Rein, T., Karri, S. K., Yakhkind, A., . . . Jensen, J. E. (2010). Effects of yoga versus walking on mood, anxiety, and brain GABA levels: A randomized controlled MRS study. *Journal of Alternative and Complementary Medicine, 16*, 1145–1152. doi:10.1089/acm.2010.0007

Tangney, J. P., Baumeister, R. F., & Boone, A. L. (2004). High self control predicts good adjustment, less pathology, better grades, and interpersonal success.*JournalofPersonality,72*,271–324.doi:10.1111/j.0022-3506.2004.00263.x

Taras, H. (2005). Physical activity and student performance at school. *Journal of School Health, 75*, 214–218.

Telles, S., Singh, N., Joshi, M., & Balkrishna, A. (2010). Post traumatic stress symptoms and heart rate variability in Bihar flood survivors following yoga: A randomized controlled study. *BMC Psychiatry, 10*(1), 18. doi:10.1186/1471-244X-10-18

Templin, S. (2015). How do I quiet my busy anxious mind: Simply notice. Retrieved from http://stevetemplin.com/how-do-i-quiet-my-busy-anxious-mind/

Thoms, S. (2011, February 28). Experts agree that laughter, humor speed up healing. *Michigan Live.* Retrieved from http://www.mlive.com/health/index .ssf/2011/02/experts_agree_that_laughter_hu.html

Toland, S. (2014, July 3). Beyond downward dog: The rise of yoga in the NBA and other pro sports. *Sports Illustrated.* Retrieved from http://www.si.com /edge/2014/06/27/rise-yoga-nba-and-other-pro-sports

Tortora, G., & Grabowski, S. (1996). *Principles of anatomy and physiology.* New York: HarperCollins.

Tresniowski, A. (2005). The girl who can't feel pain. *People, 63*(3). Retrieved from http://www.people.com/people/archive/article/0,,20146647,00.html

Tyrka, A. R., Burgers, D. E., Philip, N. S., Price, L. H., & Carpenter, L. L. (2013). The neurobiological correlates of childhood adversity and implications for treatment. *Acta Psychiatrica Scandinavica, 128*(6), 434–447. doi:10.1111/acps.12143

Tyrka, A. R., Price, L. H., Marsit, C., Walters, O. C., & Carpenter, L. L. (2012). Childhood adversity and epigenetic modulation of the leukocyte glucocorticoid receptor: Preliminary findings in healthy adults. *PLoS ONE, 7*, 1.

U.S. Department of Education, Office of Special Education Programs. (2015). Positive behavioral interventions and supports: School. Retrieved from https://www.pbis.org/school

University of Texas at Dallas Student Counseling Center. (2016). Test anxiety. Retrieved from http://www.utdallas.edu/counseling/testanxiety/

Upledger Institute. (2016). Upledger Institute International: Discover craniosacral therapy. Retrieved from http://upledger.com/therapies/index.php

van der Kolk, B. (2014). *The body keeps the score: Brain, mind, and body in the healing of trauma.* New York: Viking.

van der Kolk, B. A., Stone, L., West, J., Rhodes, A., Emerson, D., Suvak, M., & Spinazzola, J. (2014). Yoga as an adjunctive treatment for posttraumatic stress disorder: A randomized controlled trial. *Journal of Clinical Psychiatry, 75*(6), 559–565. doi:10.4088/JCP.13m08561

Van de Weijer-Bergsma, E., Formsma, A. R., de Bruin, E. I., & Bögels, S. M. (2012). The effectiveness of mindfulness training on behavioral problems and attentional functioning in adolescents with ADHD. *Journal of Child and Family Studies, 21*(5), 775–787. http://doi.org/10.1007/s10826-011-9531-7

Vaughn, S., & Fuchs, L. S. (2003). Redefining learning disabilities as inadequate response to instruction: The promise and potential problems. *Learning Disabilities Research and Practice, 18,* 137–146.

Villemure, C., Ceko, M., Cotton, V. A., & Bushnell, M. C. (2013). Insular cortex mediates increased pain tolerance in yoga practitioners. *Cerebral Cortex, 24*, 2732–2740. doi:10.1093/cercor/bht124

Vishnudevananda, S. (1960). *The complete illustrated book of yoga.* New York: Harmony.

Vythilingam, M., Heim, C., Newport, J., Miller, A., Anderson, E., Bronen, R. M., &

Bremner, J. (2002). Childhood trauma associated with smaller hippocampi in women with major depression. *American Journal of Psychiatry, 159*, 2072–2080.

Walsh, D. (2012, Winter). The brain goes to school. Paper presented at Learning and the Brain 31st Conference, San Francisco, CA.

Weare, K. (2015). Innovative contemplative/mindfulness based approaches to mental health in schools. In S. Kutcher, Y. Wei Y, & M. Weist (Eds.), *School mental health: Global opportunities and challenges* (pp. 252–266). Cambridge: Cambridge University Press.

Weintraub, A. (2004). *Yoga for depression*. New York: Broadway.

Weintraub, A. (2012). *Yoga skills for therapists*. New York: Norton.

Wenig, M. (2003). *YogaKids: Educating the Whole Child through Yoga*. New York: Stewart, Tabori, and Chang.

White, D. G. (1996). *The alchemical body: Siddha traditions in medieval India*. Chicago: University of Chicago Press.

White, D. G. (2014). *The yoga sutra of Patanjali: A biography*. Princeton, NJ: Princeton University Press.

Williams, A. K. (2000). *Being black: Zen and the art of living with fearlessness and grace*. New York: Penguin.

Willis, J. (2008). *How your child learns best.* Naperville, IL: Sourcebooks.

Willis, J. (2014, July 18). The neuroscience behind stress and learning. Edutopia, Brain-Based Learning. Retrieved from http://www.edutopia.org/blog/neuro science-behind-stress-and-learning-judy-willis

Wong, K. (2011, November 23). Adam Levine give details about his routine before concerts. Hollyscoop. Retrieved from http://edit.stage.hollyscoop .com/adam-levine/adam-levine-gives-details-about-his-routine-before -concerts.html

Woodyard, C. (2011). Exploring the therapeutic effects of yoga and its ability to increase quality of life. *International Journal of Yoga, 4*(2), 49–54. http://doi. org/10.4103/0973-6131.85485

Woolery, A., Myers, H., Sternlieb, B., & Zeltzer, L. (2004). A yoga intervention for young adults with elevated symptoms of depression. *Alternative Therapies in Health and Medicine, 10*, 60–63.

World Health Organization. (2009). Children and noise. Retrieved from http:// www.who.int/ceh/capacity/noise.pdf

Yoga Calm. (2007). School yoga research. Retrieved from http://www.yoga calm.org/about/research

Young, E. (2001). Balancing act. *New Scientist*, *15*, 25.

Zenner, C., Herrnleben-Kurz, S., & Walach, H. (2014, June 30). Mindfulness-based interventions in schools—a systematic review and meta-analysis. *Frontiers in Psychology*. http://dx.doi.org/10.3389/fpsyg.2014.00603

Zimmerman, R. (2014, April 10). Newton deploys relaxation experts to help de-stress community. WBUR's Common Health: Reform and Reality. Retrieved from http://commonhealth.wbur.org/2014/04/newton-deploys-relaxation-experts-to-help-de-stress-community

Zurchin, C. (2015). Kripalu yoga in schools symposium 2015. Kripalu Center for Yoga and Health. Lenox, MA

Zylowska, L., Ackerman, D. L., Yang, M. H., Futrell, J. L., Horton, N. L., Hale, T. S., Pataki, C., & Smalley, S. L. (2008). Mindfulness meditation training in adults and adolescents with ADHD: A feasibility study. *Journal of Attention Disorders, 11*(6), 737–746.

Yoga Programs Cited in *Classroom Yoga Breaks: Brief Exercises to Create Calm*

Bent on Learning, http://bentonlearning.org/

Breathe First Curriculum, http://www.breathefirstcurriculum.com

Classroom Yoga Breaks, http://www.classroomyogabreaks.com

Creative Relaxation Yoga, http://www.creativerelaxationyoga.com; http://www.yogaforspecialneeds.com/

Grounded Kids Yoga, http://www.gogrounded.com/

Headstand, http://www.headstand.org/

Himalayan Institute, https://www.himalayaninstitute.org/

Holistic Life Foundation, http://hlfinc.org/

International Sivananda Yoga Vedanta Centres, http://www.sivananda.org/

K–12YOGA: International Association for School Yoga and Mindfulness, http://k-12yoga.org/

Kidding Around Yoga, http://kiddingaroundyoga.com/

Kripalu Center for Yoga and Health, https://kripalu.org/

Kripalu Yoga in the Schools Teacher Training, https://kripalu.org/kyis-teacher-training

Laughter Yoga, http://www.laughteryoga.org/english/home

Learning to Breathe, http://learning2breathe.org/

Lineage Project, http://*www.lineageproject.org/*

Little Flower Yoga, http://littlefloweryoga.com

Mindful Practices, http://www.mindfulpracticesyoga.com/

Move Through Yoga, http://www.movethroughyoga.com/

National Kids Yoga Conference, www.kidsyogaconference.org

Newark Yoga Movement, http://www.newarkyogamovement.org/

1000 Petals, http://www.1000-petals.com/

Peace in Schools, http://www.peaceinschools.org/

S.T.O.P. and Relax, http://www.stopandrelaxyoga.com

The Connection Coalition, http://www.theconnectioncoalition.org/

Theoyoga, http://www.theoga.net/

Yoga Calm, http://www.yogacalm.org/

Yoga Ed, http://yogaed.com/

Yoga 4 Classrooms, http://www.yoga4classrooms.com/

Yoga Gangsters, http://yogagangsters.org/

Yoga in Schools, http://yogainschools.org/

YogaKids, http://yogakids.com/

Yoga Therapy for Children with Autism and Special Needs, http://yogaforspecialneeds.com

Yogis in Service, http://www.yogisinservice.org

Zensational Kids, http://zensationalkids.com/

Index